To my dear friend
Wishing you h
Joyce

THE CHRONIC DISEASE/POLLUTION CONNECTION

HOW TO STOP THE SPREAD OF CHRONIC DISEASE CLUSTERS

by
Joyce L. Hansel

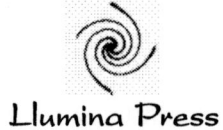

Llumina Press

Disclaimer

Information in this book is derived from my personal experiences, public records, published studies, research data, and media reports. No information in this book should be misconstrued in any way as legal or medical advice.

© 2005 Joyce L. Hansel

All rights reserved. No part of this publication may be reproduced or transmitted in any form or by any means electronic or mechanical, including photocopy, recording, or any information storage and retrieval system, without permission in writing from both the copyright owner and the publisher.

Requests for permission to make copies of any part of this work should be mailed to Permissions Department, Llumina Press, PO Box 772246, Coral Springs, FL 33077-2246

ISBN: 1-59526-033-1 PB
      1-59526-034-X HC

Printed in the United States of America by Llumina Press

Library of Congress Control Number: 2005905184

Dedication

I dedicate this book to my granddaughter Brittany, in hopes that she, her generation, and future generations can live in a cleaner, healthier environment.

About The Author

The author is a Registered Nurse who found herself living in the midst of a Multiple Sclerosis disease cluster in a quaint village in Ohio. Soon she was also diagnosed with MS and forced to retire from a successful nursing career. Still she feels that some good came out of her forced retirement. It helped her look at the U.S. health care system outside the confines of a hospital. What she found shocked and concerned her and caused her to write to warn others about how their health may be affected by living in areas of past or continuing pollution. More importantly, she gives insights into how our public health system can be improved, and where readers can get information to better understand how their environment can be improved by cleaning up past pollution and reducing the generation of further pollution.

She is a graduate of Diploma School of Nursing and University BSN Program. Her nursing career spans over 30 years in nursing and hospital supervision positions as well as a college Clinical Nursing Instructor.

Contents

Introduction		i
Chapter 1	The Wellington, Ohio MS Disease Cluster	1
Chapter 2	Surprising High Incidence of Chronic Disease Clusters	11
Chapter 3	Toxic Chemicals in Our Environment	15
Chapter 4	U.S. Failure to Stop Polluting Industries	27
Chapter 5	Power Plants, Toxic Waste Incinerators and Nuclear Plants	39
Chapter 6	Environmental Protection Agency (EPA)	45
Chapter 7	Brownfields	49
Chapter 8	U.S.EPA Authority and Superfund Sites	57
Chapter 9	Heavy Metal Poisoning in the U.S	61
Chapter 10	Mercury Contamination	69
Chapter 11	Cancer and the Environmental Connection	73
Chapter 12	Asbestos and Silica Exposure Problems	81
Chapter 13	Childhood Disease Clusters - Asthma	91
Chapter 14	Childhood Disease Clusters - Cancer	95
Chapter 15	Childhood Disease Clusters - Birth Defects	103
Chapter 16	The Military Base/Disease Cluster Connection	109
Chapter 17	Many Other Disease Clusters	113
Chapter 18	Why Disease Cluster Studies Fail	123
Chapter 19	Mistakes Made and Lessons Learned By Disease Cluster Health Advocates	135
Bibliography		137

Appendix A	Guide to Finding Help for Your Community's Environmental Health Problems	147
Appendix B	Glossary of Acronyms	153
Appendix C	Health Effects of the Most Toxic Substances Found at Superfund Sites	157

Introduction

The village of Wellington, Ohio, where my husband and I raised our three sons, was peaceful and virtually crime-free. It seemed like an ideal place to live until I found myself living in the midst of a Multiple Sclerosis (MS) disease cluster. Call it fate, or coincidence, or just bad luck. I was also diagnosed with MS, and it gradually progressed to the point that made working very difficult. I had been employed for more than thirty years as a registered nurse before being forced to retire in 1996. It was an uncomfortable transition from caregiver to the one needing care, but I feel that some positives came out of my diagnosis and forced retirement. For one, it made me look at our nation's health care system outside the confines of a hospital. What I learned was very surprising and left me shaking my head in disbelief.

The increasing incidence of chronic disease is alarming and reason for concern. The causes of most chronic diseases are unknown and often occur in concentrated geographical areas, or clusters. The medical profession defines chronic diseases as diseases lasting a long time, reoccurring often, and resisting efforts to eradicate them. This is in contrast to a communicable or infectious disease that can be transmitted from person to person and has a known cause and cure. A disease cluster is usually defined as a number of people with the same disease living in close proximity to each other. Disease clusters are almost always found in an area of toxic pollution from nearby industry. There are laws to stop polluters, but state and federal agencies often fail to enforce them. The lack of enforcement is all too often because of political and special interest pressures, and always to the detriment to peoples' health.

I have learned hard lessons from what happened in my community and hope to give you the information needed to understand the magnitude of the problems, and the need to become proactive to protect the health of your family and neighborhoods. When I looked for other chronic disease clusters I found them occurring across the nation. **We have chronic diseases occurring at epidemic rates.**

Accurate statistical data regarding the actual incidence of a chronic disease is often not available. Also there is no fully-operational national disease tracking network. This is a major problem that you will hear about often in this book and in the media. The following information was available from several public health advocacy organizations and the government.

- The Center for Disease Control and Prevention (CDC) reports that "7 out of 10 Americans die each year from chronic diseases. More than 1.7 million people will die each year from chronic diseases. One in 10 Americans has a disabling condition."
- Asthma increased 75% between 1980 and 1994. Asthma is the most common childhood disease. More than seventeen million Americans suffer from asthma. Experts predicted that the number would double in the following twenty years
- Multiple sclerosis rates rose 20% between 1986 and 1995. Over 300,000 people are diagnosed with MS in the United States today.

Introduction

- The number of lupus cases in the United States is estimated to be 1,500,000. Lupus deaths among African American women between 45 and 64 years of age increased 70% in a twenty year period.
- Elevated birth defect rates are occurring across the country in areas with toxic pollution. The CDC reports that birth defects are the leading cause of death in the first year of life. About 120,000 babies are born each year with birth defects and 8,000 die during their first year of life."
- The American Cancer Society's "Cancer Facts and Figures 2005" predicts that "1,372,910 new cases of cancer will be diagnosed in 2005 and 570,280 Americans are expected to die of cancer, more than 1500 people per day."

This book contains information about why chronic disease cluster studies fail to identify causes for the clustering of a chronic disease. You will also learn about the weaknesses in our public health system and what is needed to bring about change. **Development of chronic disease clusters is preventable!**

Looking into other disease clusters, I found a lack of action by both affected residents and the health care agencies paid to protect them. You may not be aware of how much pollution is in your neighborhoods, but you can easily find out when you know the government and environmental group sources for information. When you know the laws, you can pressure state and federal agencies to act. **Toxic pollution can be controlled!**

Hearing about some chronic disease clusters and their connection to polluting industries should paint a good picture about what is happening in our communities. Let me start first with the story of my Wellington MS disease cluster.

| Introduction

Please note the quick references in appendix B for acronyms (those capital letters used to identify organizations) and appendix C for a list of toxic chemicals and their effects on our bodies.

Chapter 1

The Wellington Ohio MS Disease Cluster

Wellington is a community full of quaint, well-kept historical homes, as well as subdivisions of new modern homes. There is a town square with a park, a gazebo, and an operating town hall built in 1885. It is a typical small town, with a population of less than 5,000 people, where most everyone seems to know everyone else. But it took many years for people to recognize an eerie presence just a few blocks from that town square. Neighbors were discussing fatigue, numbness, and weakness in their feet and legs. Some people were having trouble with balance and walking. You could stand on a street and point out houses where people were being diagnosed with neurological problems.

It was obvious that the people with neurological problems were clustered within about a sixth block area. Something was very wrong for so many people, living in such a small area, to all have neurological problems! Alarm spread from neighbor to neighbor, and in 1984 a support group was organized called "Citizens for a Clean Environment." They counted thirty two ill people at that time. Eight affected people lived on Prospect Street alone. Two children who spent their summers with their grandparents on Prospect Street throughout their school years were both diagnosed with MS as young adults, but are not included in the count since their home was not in Wellington.

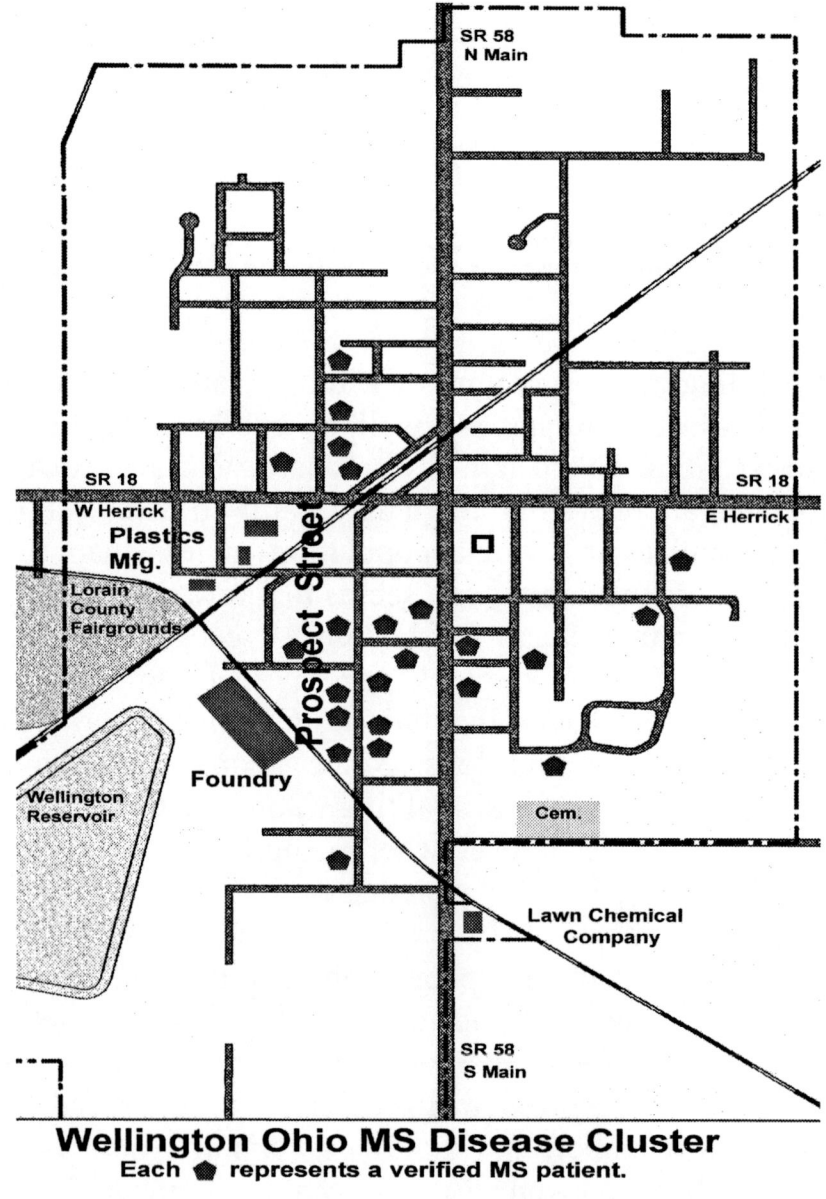

Wellington Ohio MS Disease Cluster
Each ⬟ represents a verified MS patient.

Was it something in the water, the air, the soil? Support group members would get together and try to support each other. They would discuss the possible courses of action to take to get answers for the many MS cases. The support group took the obvious first step and contacted our Lorain County Health Department (LCHD). Eventually, the LCHD sent questionnaires to the group, which were quickly filled out and returned. They waited for the next step but heard nothing. Sometime later a support group member called the health department to see what else would be done and was told that there was no funding for any kind of the study in Wellington. If your health department can't help you, what could you do next?

Everyone in the support group was discouraged. Attending meetings was difficult because of increasing impairment of cluster members, so attendance slowly dwindled. They were trying to live with the hopeless diagnoses, while attempting to hold on to their jobs and maintain their households. This was especially discouraging because MS has no known cause or cure, and the rate of progression of the disease is unpredictable.

Years passed quickly and the health of people in the disease cluster deteriorated at different rates. This is typical of MS because it is a disease of remissions and exacerbations (flare-ups). Getting a diagnosis is difficult and usually takes years. Symptoms include numbness and weakness in the extremities, problems with vision and cognition, urinary difficulties, gradual loss of mobility, minimal to severe nerve pain in various parts of the body, and overwhelming fatigue. Some people in the disease cluster found it necessary to use canes, some walkers, and others wheelchairs. MS is not considered a terminal illness. People usually die from complications from impaired mobility, loss of neurological function, or another chronic disease. While some people can live a long life, others progress rapidly and have a short life span.

The disease cluster group continued to search for reasons for the MS disease cluster and it seemed reasonable to focus on the environment. Something in the six block area that they shared must be making people sick. The three most obvious sources of possible environmental contamination were a foundry that produced iron castings, a plastics manufacturer, and a fertilizer manufacturer.

Most families suspected that the foundry was the source of our problems, because of its longstanding practice of expelling large amounts of fine red ashes from its tall smoke stack, usually at night. Red ashes frequently covered houses and automobiles in the area of the factory. The amounts were such that residents were often required to perform daily cleanups to their homes and automobiles. Families living near the foundry spoke of a frequent very strong odor like burning wires. Wellington residents reportedly sent fifty one complaints about the problems to the Ohio Environmental Protection Agency (OEPA) over a nine year period. To our knowledge, not one resident ever received a response from the OEPA during that time. The affected Wellington residents concluded that, once again, the agencies paid to protect us failed to do so. First it was the LCHD and now it was the OEPA.

A few people continued to fight to find a reason for Wellington's MS disease cluster. Most people stopped participating in what they saw as a futile fight, and our support group dwindled to three members. One particular cluster member, Sally, continues to live in the midst of the MS disease cluster and never gave up hope of finding a reason for so many sick people in her neighborhood. Marilyn and I joined Sally in the continuing search for answers. Marilyn doesn't have MS, but she too is searching for answers since her daughter Terri is an affected member of the MS disease cluster. Terri is a beautiful young woman who was a popular prom queen at Wellington High School. She was looking forward to a happy, productive life. But after her marriage and the birth of her two children, she was stricken with MS at age twenty three. She and her husband were soon divorced and her husband moved away with their children. Terri's MS progressed rapidly and she soon required assistance with most activities of daily living. She chose to move into a facility in a town near her children so that she could see them as much as possible. Marilyn has remained very involved in Terri's life and has been Terri's biggest supporter.

Our small support group continued to contact public health officials, as well as our government representatives. Then, in March 1999, a nearby city newspaper reporter wrote a series of articles about the MS disease cluster in Wellington. The reporter met with and interviewed disease cluster members and physicians in the area. The published reports provided a detailed series of articles that won a well-deserved journalism award. It also garnered national attention to the health problems in Wellington. It is frustrating to think that it took a series of newspaper articles to get someone to respond to citizens' concerns. Wellington residents had been asking for help since 1984. Fifteen years is a long time for people to wait who are ill or becoming ill with a higher than normal occurrence of a disease. (I had no idea that it would eventually become twenty years and there would still be no answers).

Then we got a break! Sally had been in contact with individuals at the Agency for Toxic Substances and Disease

Registry (ATSDR), which is part of the U.S. Department of Health & Human Services. The ATSDR "evaluates environmental and health outcome data to determine the possible health effects of exposure to hazardous substances. They work with local, state and other federal agencies to protect public health by preventing and reducing these types of exposure." In November 1999, Sally was invited to speak about the Wellington disease cluster at the American Public Health Association meeting in Chicago. Then, in June 2000, the ATSDR informed Sally that federal funds were available to determine the prevalence of MS in communities living near hazardous waste sites. Sally gave the information to the LCHD and the Ohio Department of Health (ODH) who both applied for and received funding. They needed funding and Sally got them funding! We were thrilled that now someone would finally look into our health problems in Wellington.

The LCHD investigated and confirmed twenty three cases of MS in Wellington. They did this by reviewing medical records and consulting with the neurologists of disease cluster members. Several disease cluster members had moved away and some had died, so their data was not included. The LCHD told us that there were insufficient funds or personnel to contact people who had moved to other communities.

Several people who thought they may have had MS were diagnosed with lupus, a chronic inflammatory disease causing abnormalities in blood vessels and connective tissue. The MS Society determined that, according to their statistics, the number of cases of MS in our disease cluster was five times higher than it should be for a population of less than 5000 people.

Our optimism about having a study performed for our MS cluster was short-lived. We soon learned that the federal funds were for the purpose of developing the methodology and procedures for doing an MS health study, not for doing an actual study in Wellington. One would think that the methodology and procedures for doing a health study would be covered in Epidemiology 101, but that is apparently not the case with MS and most other chronic diseases. These federal funds were being provided for a cooperative Prevalence Study among three states with MS disease clusters. The three areas were Lorain County, Ohio; Independence and Sugar Creek Missouri, and a nineteen county area surrounding Lubbock, Texas.

Independence and Sugar Creek, with a combined population of 120,000 people, reported a two-to-four-fold number of cases of MS above what should be expected. The Lubbock, Texas area was reported to be included because it did not have a suspected high number of MS cases and would be used to establish the norm.

We were disappointed again to learn that ODH would not do a Prevalence Study just in Wellington, but would expand the Ohio study to include all MS cases in Lorain County. Wouldn't that take the focus off of our disease cluster in Wellington? Would the results not change if we were lumped into the approximately 280,000 population in the County? The Chief of Chronic & Environmental Disease Surveillance Section at the ODH assured us that this would not be the case. Expanding the study area has been done before in ODH studies and in studies performed in other states. However, public health and environmental support organization critics say this dilutes the significance of the disease cluster. How could it not make a difference?

Since we still feared that our Wellington MS disease cluster would be ignored, we continued to look for someone to examine our unique cluster of twenty three confirmed MS cases in a six block area. I wrote letters asking for advice and help from government officials, the US Department of Health and Human Services, and other government agencies involved in U.S. health programs. Sometimes I received a response, but often it was a generic response that acknowledged the contact. I later learned that asking your elected government representatives to contact state and federal public health agencies about your concerns makes it more likely that your request will be addressed.

Then we learned that the ATSDR could do a health consultation of a disease cluster if the site was determined to be a possible threat to public health. We wrote a letter to the ATSDR in March 2003 requesting a health consultation in Wellington. We were unsure if our disease cluster would qualify, but we soon learned that we did indeed qualify for further investigation.

On September 5, 2003 an ATSDR representative visited Wellington and consulted with the OEPA and the ODH. Later the same day, she met with several members of our disease cluster, together with representatives from the LCHD and the ODH. We were told that an ATSDR health consultation involved reviewing and summarizing available data, considering public health implications, and making public health recommendations. Additional exposure related data would be collected if it were needed. The ODH would work with ATSDR in their consultation. At our meeting we discussed the fact that many years have now passed and that the foundry recently closed its doors and quietly left town. The fertilizer company's buildings were being used for storage only, and the plastics factory has long met EPA standards. We were told that if a study had been done looking at these facilities years ago, we could be more optimistic about finding toxic substances in the environment or a reason for our illnesses. I couldn't help but feel anger when I heard this. By then it had been 20 years since we started asking for help.

Then the ODH also announced that they would be doing MS Case Control Studies in Wellington. Disease cluster members have been asked to sign permits for the study and for blood work. I have not been contacted to participate which raises a question in my mind about how accurate this study can be if not everyone was included. Although we thought the case studies would involve only the Wellington disease cluster members, again we learned that the studies would include all of the Lorain County population as well as the same Missouri and Texas groups that were involved in that first (Prevalence) study. Once again Wellington was being lumped into an expanded population.

In the spring of 2003, I contacted the ODH to ask when the results of the Prevalence Study would be announced. The study was to have been completed in two years but it was then over three years. I was told that results were delayed because of the need to include nursing home patients in Lorain County who have MS. I was also told that results so far found the number of MS cases in Lorain County to be significantly higher than expected and that Wellington was "unique." The number mentioned for Lorain County Ms cases was 271 cases at that time. I was told results would be out in a few weeks. Still, in mid June 2005 no results of the Prevalence Study have been reported.

Our hope is that any remaining toxic substances in the area (especially in the foundry's eight acre dump site) can be identified and compared to other MS disease cluster findings.

Then, perhaps common findings could at least point to a possible disease trigger. Also, we want to be sure that our community is safe for the many families who are now building homes in new subdivisions near the disease cluster area.

Will we ever learn why Wellington has an MS disease cluster of people residing in a six block area? Reading research articles and public health studies involving other disease clusters convinced me that it is doubtful that we will learn much, if anything. Public Health official are quoted as saying "that it is hard to say that a certain toxic exposure in a neighborhood caused a chronic disease cluster, since the cause of the disease is usually unknown." Critics say that public health studies of disease clusters are designed to fail. I don't know if that is true of all states. We can only hope that this was not the case with our ODH.

Chapter 2

Surprising High Incidence of Chronic Disease Clusters

I wanted to find out more about MS disease clusters, so I turned to the internet. I searched government reports, research reports and media stories for more information. I found a lot of information about MS disease clusters. However I also found chronic disease clusters of all types of cancer, Parkinson's disease, autism, birth defects, fibromyalgia, lupus, Alzheimer's disease, asthma, and in fact just about every chronic disease known to man. It looked like a chronic disease epidemic to me, but how can one know for sure? There is no way of knowing how many people are sick or where they are located throughout a state or throughout the nation.

I learned, from archived newspaper reports, that there was an MS disease cluster in a small town just thirty five miles south of Wellington in Ashland County. At the same time I learned of another MS disease cluster in Lorain, Ohio, just twenty miles north of Wellington. Lorain had a reported disease cluster of at least eight cases of MS in the Lorain High School 1980 graduating class of three hundred fifty students. Prior to doing the media searches, I had no idea they existed.

| How To Stop the Spread of Chronic Disease Clusters

One disease cluster is usually unaware of any other disease cluster unless they learn about it in the news media. Local health departments learn about a disease cluster from members of a disease cluster or someone living in the disease cluster area. State health departments learn about a disease cluster the same way, or the local health department reports the problem to them. The CDC is the last to know, and then only if state officials notify them. What is desperately needed is a comprehensive country-wide disease tracking network. This disease tracking network could then locate the disease clusters quickly, start studies quickly, compare common findings, and possibly discover disease triggers. This could lead to finding causes and cures for chronic diseases. The need for this system has been advocated by dozens of environmental and public health support groups for years now. Later chapters will include more on this topic.

My search for other MS disease clusters located many more other types of chronic disease clusters than I could imagine. I soon had so much information it became difficult to remember the information accurately. Then I began making written notes and printing the information and organizing it in folders. It became increasingly important to me to warn people about the many disease clusters in our neighborhoods and their connection to pollution.

It seemed that the media was the appropriate source to get my message to the most people. I contacted local newspapers, TV stations, and radio stations. Due to my efforts I was able to report my concerns during a short interview with a small local radio station and a Cleveland television station. When the television report was aired it included one brief statement from me taken out of context. It seemed like a good plan but it failed to get my message to the public.

After about 18 months, I realized that I had more than enough information to write a book. And, I felt that writing such a book would probably reach the many other people who have had or are having clusters of chronic health problems. Many are living in the shadows of polluting industries, yet unaware of toxins in their air and water.

Chapter 3

Toxic Chemicals in Our Environment

Disease clusters are almost always located near polluted land, air, or water. Sadly, many communities are often dealing with all three sources. Toxic chemicals are all around us but we can not easily see that they are invading our neighborhoods. Each year industrial facilities nationwide release millions of pounds of toxic chemicals into our air and water. These chemicals are linked to cancer, neurological and respiratory disorders, and to developmental and reproductive problems. Yet, communities living in the shadow of the industrial facilities typically are unaware of the pollution in their backyards. To get a good picture of what is occurring, I will try to explain how this country manages toxic chemicals.

The Federal Toxic Release Inventory

The U.S.EPA manages the Toxics Release Inventory (TRI) which contains data on toxic chemical releases and other waste management information. The TRI report is published to inform the public about chemical releases in the environment. Activities reported annually cover toxic releases by certain industry groups as well as federal facilities. The TRI was established under the Emergency Planning and Community Right-to-Know Act of 1986 and expanded by the Pollution Prevention Act of 1990.

The toxic chemical amounts are alarming! Yet the TRI covers only about 1% of the 80,000 chemicals in commercial use today. The report only covers releases from the largest industries, with information provided by the industries themselves. This appears to be the best government data available on toxic releases.

Toxic Chemical Release Research

The PennEnvironment Research and Policy Center, and the U.S Public Interest Research Group (US PIRG) evaluated the TRI data and explained the impact on public health of the chemical releases. The 2003 report is titled "Toxic Releases and Health, A Review of Pollution Data and the Current Knowledge on the Health Effects of Toxic Chemicals." We should be very grateful to organizations like these two for looking out for us and our environment. You will learn about more dedicated public health advocacy organizations in future chapters.

The PennEnvironment Research and Policy Center is a research and public education center. PennEnvironment's mission is "to deliver persistent, result-oriented advocacy that preserves our environment, protects the public's health, and fosters responsive, democratic government."

The U.S.PIRG mission is "to uncover threats to public health and well-being and fight to end them, using time-tested tools of investigative research, media, grassroots organizing, advocacy, and litigation."

Both the PennEnvironment and USPIRG research are well respected by environmental health advocacy groups as well as government agencies. Their research found the following regarding toxic chemical releases into America's air and water. These are the findings for <u>annual releases.</u>

- "More than one hundred million pounds of cancer-causing chemical releases.
- One hundred thirty eight million pounds of chemicals linked to birth defects and learning disabilities.
- Fifty million pounds of chemicals related to reproductive disorders.
- More than one billion pounds of suspected neurological toxicants.
- More than 1.7 billion pounds of suspected respiratory toxicants.
- More than 7000grams of dioxin, which scientists believe to be the most toxic substance in our environment."

Two other highly toxic substances that are very detrimental to health were also specifically mentioned. Lead (275,000 lbs.), lead compounds (1.3 million lbs.) and mercury (30,000 lbs) and mercury compounds (136,000 lbs.).

Lead and mercury toxicity will be discussed in detail later.

The Toxic Substance Control Act

In 1976 the Toxic Substance Control Act was enacted by Congress to help manage the increasing numbers of industrial chemicals produced or imported into the United States. There were 55,000 chemicals in use when the Act became law. The Act includes measures to control exposure to asbestos, lead, and radon. The toxic effects of these chemicals and the number of disease clusters connected to these chemicals could not be ignored. But as of this writing, the EPA still had no toxicity data or safe levels for most chemicals in the environment. The EPA task is a huge one and they may be doing the best they can with the resources available.

The majority of the public still believes that chemicals are completely tested by the government. Unfortunately, this is not the case. As mentioned earlier, chemical companies do their own testing and submit the results to the EPA for review, thus setting up the potential for selective reporting.

Another problem is the number of new chemicals introduced into our environment each year. As mentioned earlier, U.S. chemical companies hold licenses to make about 80,000 chemicals for commercial use and the government on average registers an additional 2,000 chemicals yearly. These chemicals are the ingredients for our cosmetics, preservatives, and additives in foods, consumer products, and pesticides. We need to use some chemicals in our environment but overuse creates serious problems. One example is pesticides

Pesticides

There are great concerns about the overuse of pesticides in this country. Farmers often overuse chemicals to kill off weeds and crop diseases. Home owners often overuse chemicals on their lawns to have greener, weed-free lawns. Common pesticides used in the home and yard are believed to be responsible for children's' learning disabilities, respiratory conditions, mental retardation, and damage to the immune and nervous systems. Developing fetuses, infants and young children are most susceptible to toxic chemicals.

Chronic Disease / Pollution Connection

The number of cases of asthma has increased dramatically in the last twenty years in both adults and children, and this is believed to be from exposure to chemicals and pesticides used in and around the home.

In May, 2003 a school in northeastern Ohio reported that an exterminator sprayed chemicals around a middle school that sent one teacher home and forty two students to the hospital.

The following information on pesticides was taken from a report written by Nathan Diegelman from the 'Sensitive To A Toxic Environment' Foundation (S.T.A.T.E.) and is titled "Poison in the Grass: The Hazards and Consequences of Lawn Pesticides."

The report is shocking, to say the least! Here are a few highlights from Dr. Diegelman's report.

"Pesticides engulf the home and are easily tracked inside, readily inhaled and absorbed through the skin. They do harm by attacking the central nervous system and other essential organs. Symptoms of pesticide poisoning are often deceptively simple and are commonly misdiagnosed as flu or allergies.

According to the EPA, 95% of the pesticides used on residential lawns are possible or probable carcinogens - - -. In 1989 the National Cancer Institute reported children develop leukemia six times more often when pesticides are used around their homes - - -. The American Journal of Epidemiology found that more children with brain tumors and other cancers had been exposed to insecticides than children without. - - - Studies by the National Cancer Society and other medical researchers have discovered a definite link between fatal non-Hodgkins Lymphoma (NHL) and exposure to triazine herbicides (like Atrazine), phenoxyacetic herbicides (2,4-D), organophosphate insecticides (Diazinon), fungicides, and fumigants; all of which have uses as lawn chemicals. This may be an important contributing factor to the 50% rise in NHL over the past ten years in the American population. Studies of farmers who once used these pesticides found alarmingly high numbers of NHL, especially in those who didn't wear protective clothing. This latest finding also proves the theory that most danger from pesticides comes through dermal absorption, not ingestion - - -. A University of Iowa study of golf course superintendents found abnormally high rates of death due to cancer of the brain, large intestine, and prostate. Other experts are beginning to link golfers, and non-golfers who live near fairways, with these same problems.

Chemicals applied to our lawns are most poisonous from inhaling pesticide residue or absorbing them through our skin. Pesticides and chemical fertilizers find there way into our water supplies and are becoming some of the worst water pollutants in America. Discharges of chemicals into San Francisco Bay from the central valley of California are estimated at almost two tons per year. Phosphorous levels in some Maryland streams have doubled since 1986. The EPA has found potentially harmful levels of nitrate from chemical fertilizers in drinking water wells nationwide. Agricultural and consumer purchased pesticides are not currently required to be tested for even subtle neurological effects and this is reason for concern."

Wildlife pathologists have studied animals and birds killed by pesticides that were used according to regulations. They document cases of owls, robins, doves, sparrows, cardinals, bluebirds, and many other songbirds killed by chemicals. Waterfowl like Canadian geese, mallards, wood ducks, and others have also been affected. One wildlife pathologist likens these birds to the miners' canaries, warning of danger to man.

We must become proactive in order to protect ourselves and our families from the many chemicals we are exposed to everyday. We need to educate ourselves about the ingredients found in household products and to check ingredient information on product labels when purchasing them. Don't let those long chemical names intimidate you. Become familiar with the few you see repeatedly. Be aware that there can be interactions between products used together, and always follow instructions listed on product labels. Experts recommend that consumers always wear rubber gloves and have good ventilation in the room when using cleaning products in the home.

You can find information on chemicals in products by accessing the internet, and also at most health departments and public libraries. The National Institutes of Health (NIH) has information about common household products at their web site: You will find the internet site in the bibliography in the back of the book. These are some of the headings found at the site. Choose a product on their site and a list of chemicals will be provided.

- Arts and Crafts   Adhesive, Glaze, Glue, Varnish and more.
- Auto Products   Brake Fluid, De-icer, Lubricant and more.

- Home Maintenance — Caulk, Grout, Insulation, paint, Putty, Stain, and more.
- Inside the Home — Air Freshener, Bleach, Cleansers, Toilet Bowl Cleanser, and more.
- Landscape/Yard — Fertilizer, Lawn Care, Swimming Pool Products and more.
- Personal Care/use — Antiperspirant, hair Spray, Makeup, Shampoo, Soap, and more.
- Pesticides — Animal Repellant, Fungicide, and more.
- Pet Care — Flea&Tick Control, Litter, Stain/Odor Remover and more."

The Chemical Body Burden

The <u>chemical body burden</u> refers to the total amount of chemicals that are present in the human body at any given point in time. You will be hearing more and more these days about the body burden in government as well as private research and in media reports. Some chemicals remain in the body for a short period of time before being excreted. Other chemicals can remain in the body for years, in our blood, fatty tissue, muscle, bone, brain tissue, and other body organs. Pesticides can remain in the body for fifty years. As reported earlier, we inhale chemicals, swallow them in food and water, and absorb them through our skin.

The CDC investigated the chemical body burden in 2001 for twenty seven environmental chemicals and in 2003 they studied another one hundred environmental chemicals and issued the following report to the public.

- "Children have twice the levels of chlorpyrifos and other commonly used organophosphate insecticides as do adults.
- Mexican Americans have three times the levels of the pesticide DDT as do whites and blacks.
- DDT is a global contaminant that, while long banned in the US and more recently in Mexico, continues to be used against malaria in some countries.
- Levels of the chemicals called phthalates that are found in cosmetics are higher in adults, especially African American women, while the more toxic phthalates found in soft PVC plastic products are higher in children."

It probably is frightening for people to hear that chemicals are building up in our bodies but it is our reality. It was frightening to me when I first heard about the body burden. I cannot understand why toxic pollution is allowed to be so out of control that our bodies become saturated and diseased.

In February 2005 two California senators submitted legislation that would establish a statewide, voluntary program to find out the amount of chemicals people have in their bodies through blood and urine studies. The results could provide clues to how toxic chemicals cause disease and hopefully find solutions to improve people's health. The plan is titled "The Healthy Californians' Biomonitoring Program."

Endocrine Disrupters

Sorry, there is more bad news. Scientists now recognize that some chemicals in our bodies can be endocrine disrupters. These chemicals upset the action of hormones in our bodies and negatively affect our health and ability to fight chronic diseases. The endocrine system can be disrupted by chemicals in several ways:

- Chemicals can directly stimulate or inhibit the endocrine system, causing over production or underproduction of hormones.
- Some chemicals can mimic a natural hormone and fool the body into responding to the chemical or responding at an inappropriate time.
- Other endocrine disrupting chemicals can block the effects of a hormone from certain receptors in our body.

The scientific community recognizes the impact chemicals are having on our bodies and are focusing more research into understanding the chemical body burden and endocrine disruption.

Multiple Chemical Sensitivity

People can be exposed to so many chemicals that some develop a condition called Multiple Chemical Sensitivity (MCS). It is a condition suspected to be caused by multiple chemical exposures and/or exposure over a long period of time. People can develop very dramatic symptoms and are often extremely disabled. Common symptoms are fatigue, dizziness, headaches, aching joints, heat intolerance, depression, and memory loss. I have met people with this condition and they are very sick and have a great deal of trouble performing even the basic activities of daily living.

The medical community is divided over whether MCS is a new diagnosis or not. A few of the other names for the condition are "environmental illness", "total allergy syndrome" and "sick house syndrome."

Some MCS people report being treated as if they were neurotic or mentally ill. It is very difficult to get a diagnosis and people often feel isolated. MCS support groups are presently found in North Carolina, Ohio, Northern Virginia, Maryland, New Mexico, Canada and the United Kingdom. People with suspected MCS are encouraged to find a physician with additional education in Multiple Chemical Sensitivity.

Chapter 4

U.S. Failure to Stop Polluting Industries

The U.S.EPA allows industrial facilities to dispose of chemicals in several ways.

- They can place them on the industry site in underground injection wells, landfills, surface enclosures, or by sending them off-site to other facilities.
- The off-site facilities can place the chemicals in underground injection wells, landfills, and/or surface enclosures.
- Some facilities can release toxic chemicals on-site into the air and into streams and nearby bodies of water, or to the facility's land or underground.
- Finally some facilities can use transfers to off-site dump sites.

The true extent of harm from polluting industries often cannot be determined because many communities are miles downwind from the emissions, and pollution levels received in those communities are not being measured. The same is true of communities downstream from polluting sites. Pollution often flows into streams, and rivers, then on to other communities and other states. In March, 2005, an Ohio industry was reportedly being sued by three surrounding states for toxic emissions polluting their air with chemicals expelled from their tall smoke stacks on a daily basis.

The continued dumping of hundreds of millions of pounds of toxic chemicals into our air and water points out the failure or inability of the government, including both state and federal EPA, to better protect us by pursuing and punishing polluters. The Clean Water Act and Clean Air Act were implemented to control polluting industries, that is, <u>if they were enforced.</u>

Congress passed the Clean Water Act in 1972 following a severe water quality crisis. The goal was to return all waters to swimmable and fishable conditions by 1983 and eliminate all pollutants in the water by 1985. Environmental support groups report that about 40% of all waters in this country remain unsafe for swimming and fishing.

A report from PennEnvironment Research and Policy Center in October 2002, titled, "In Gross Violation: How Polluters are Flooding Americas Waterways with Toxic Chemicals" points out the extent of the problem. The following are some highlights from the report.

> "Using previously non-public information provided by the EPA in response to a Freedom of Information Act (FOIA) request, this report builds on the findings of the Permit to Pollute. Rather than focusing on the facilities categorized by the EPA as in Significant Noncompliance for permit exceedances or paperwork violations, for the first time we analyze all major facilities exceeding the Clean

Chronic Disease / Pollution Connection

Water Act permits, reveal the type of pollutants they are discharging illegally in our waterways and detail the extent to which these facilities are exceeding effluent permit levels. We focus on permit exceedances for high hazard pollutants: toxicants known or suspected to cause cancer, reproductive and developmental disorders, and other serious non-cancer health effects. - - -

- Nationally, 5,116 major facilities (81%) exceed their Clean Air Act permit limits at least once between January 1, 1999 and December 31, 2001, including 1,768 facilities (28%) for discharging chemicals known or suspected to cause cancer and/or serious non-cancer health effects.
- Ten states and territories that allow the highest percentage of major facilities to exceed their Clean Water Act effluent permits at least once for high hazard chemicals are Puerto Rico, Ohio, Rhode Island, District of Columbia, Virgin Islands, New York, Arizona, Massachusetts, West Virginia and Indiana.
- Major facilities, on average, exceeded their effluent permit limits for high hazard chemicals by 849%, or more than eight times the legal limit, between January 1, 1999 and December 31, 2001.
- Nationally major facilities reported 1,562 instances between January 1,1999 and December 31, 2001 in which they exceed their Clean Water Act effluent permit limits for chemicals known or suspected to cause cancer and/or serious non cancer health effects by at least tenfold (1000%), and 363 instances of violations exceeding 100 fold(10,000%).

The ten states and territories that allow the greatest number of egregious permit exceedances – at least 500%, or five times, over the effluent permit limits – between January 1,1999 and December 31, 2001 for high hazard chemicals are Puerto Rico, Ohio, Pennsylvania, Texas, West Virginia, Indiana, Louisiana, Missouri, Maine and North Carolina."

The Clean Air Act goal was to develop national ambient air quality standards to protect the public health. In the examples of chronic disease clusters with polluting industries found in this book, you will learn that pollution laws were not enforced. Concessions are made to big industries, and when they are fined, the amounts of the fines are often insignificant.

PennEnvironment Research and Policy Center also released a research summary addressing air pollution, titled, "Danger in the Air: Unhealthy Levels of Air Pollution in 2003". Some information reported includes the following:

"While air quality has improved in the last three decades, half of all Americans live in counties where pollution exceeds national health standards. Most of these suffer from high levels of ozone and/or particle pollution. Ozone is the country's most pervasive air pollutant; particle pollution is the nation's deadliest air pollutant. Coal-fired plants and motor vehicles are the largest sources of the pollutants. This report is based on a comprehensive survey of environmental agencies from all 50 states and the District of Columbia, examines levels of ozone and fine particle pollution in cities and towns across the country in 2003 and finds that air pollution continues to pose a grave health threat to Americans."

The following research findings address U.S. states' involvement:

- "Ozone levels in 40 states and the District of Columbia exceed the 8-hour national health standards 4,583 times and the 1-hour standards 684 times in 187 days in 2003 - - -.
- Fine particle pollution exceeded the year-round national health standards in 20 states in 2003 - - - .
- Fine particle pollution exceeded the 24-hour national health standard 106 times on 39 days in 13 states in 2003 - - - ."

This report also included preliminary ozone data for 19 states and the District of Columbia for 2004, which like 2003, has been a relatively mild and wet summer. Yet, through the beginning of September 2004, ozone levels had exceeded the 8-hour standard 602 times and the 1-hour standard 84 times in these areas.

In November 2004, surprising research results were reported in the media across the country. California researchers presented extensive study results demonstrating a direct link between exposure to air pollution and the development of hardening of the arteries. Studies in the Los Angeles area found that the more air pollution there is around a person's home the thicker the walls of his or her carotid arteries become. Thickening of blood vessel walls is the leading cause of heart attacks and strokes. The EPA funded research at the University of Washington to study 8,700 people for ten years to further evaluate the link between people's exposure to air pollution and cardiovascular diseases.

Examples of what can happen in a community when Clean Air and Clean Water laws are not enforced can be found in Louisiana and Utah.

Calcasieu Parish, Louisiana

Calcasieu Parish, Louisiana may be one of the top toxic sites in the United States. It borders the Texas state line on the west side and its southern border is just a few miles from the Gulf of Mexico.

In the 1940s, Calcasieu Parish became the location for some of the nation's major oil and gas refineries. Later, they had a high concentration of petrochemical industrial facilities and vinyl manufacturers. There were dozens of industrial factories in the parish, and more than forty of these plants were located within a ten mile radius.

Industries in Calcasieu Parish were reported to annually pollute the environment with more than 9,000,000 lbs of toxic chemicals. According to surveys, the community of Morrisville in the Calcasieu Parish suffered from illnesses related to chemical exposures at a rate three times higher than that of a control group, and in every one of the twelve body system categories.

The ATSDR conducted a public health assessment in the Parish in 1999. Blood studies found dioxin blood levels that were three times higher than the national average.

The Louisiana State Health Department looked into cancer rates in the area from 1988 to 1997, and the results found the overall cancer rates to be what would be expected for a community that size. Still, the study found elevated lung cancer and soft tissue cancers. The studies failed to recognize a toxic pollution/disease connection.

When I searched to get more information on pollution in Calcasieu Parish, I found that the Parish was listed among the dirtiest counties in the country in 2002.

By the late 1990s, residents in Calcasieu Parish became disgusted by the inaction on the part of state and federal environmental agencies when they complained about the pungent odors, frequent accidents at facilities, and adverse health effects. Residents formed a cooperative training program with help from Communities for a Better Environment, an environmental support group based in California. In September, 1998 the residents began to monitor air quality on their own. The citizens' called their air monitoring effort the Bucket Brigade, after the bucket-like equipment used to obtain the air samples. They took samples following EPA protocols for handling, documenting, and delivering samples to an EPA approved laboratory for analysis. Toxic chemicals were found to be far above the state health/air quality standards. The samplings proved that industries were not controlling their emissions.

Armed with their lab results, the citizen group was able to get the EPA to increase enforcement of environmental laws. The amounts of toxic chemical releases decreased dramatically. The number of toxic release accidents decreased a great deal, although they still occurred. The citizens' Bucket Brigade and the environmental support group, Communities for a Better Environment, are among our unsung heroes in the battle for a cleaner environment.

People have lived in toxic environments like this for decades, in fact for generations, without actively seeking change. They somehow believed that the industries and public health agencies would stop industrial pollution if they could. But in the case of Calcasieu Parish, little was being done until concerned citizens became proactive in protecting their community from excessive toxic pollution.

Tooele County, Utah

Tooele County, Utah has a long toxic environment history with elevated rates of cancer, cardiac disease, asbestos related diseases, neurological diseases, and birth defects. Thirty nine cases of cancer were reported in a St. George neighborhood. Fourteen cases of MS were reported within a two-block area of another neighborhood. Tooele County was home to the nation's only commercial low-level radioactive waste dump, as well as a hazardous waste dump, and a waste incinerator. The military incinerator in Tooele County was being used to destroy massive stockpiles of chemical and biological weapons. In Granville there were reported clusters of birth defects and cancer in a town of 4400 people.

The ATSDR performed a Public Health Assessment in Tooele County and provided more information on the problems. "The site is a reclaimed mine, mill, and smelting property. Copper and lead smelting conducted there between 1910 and 1972 resulted in elevated levels of arsenic, cadmium, and lead in the soil. In 1986, the site was placed on the National Priority List for Cleanup. Contamination in the area was attributed to long-standing practices of mismanagement of waste and emissions." According to the ATSDR, people were exposed to contaminants in three ways:

1. "Ingesting or inhaling contaminated smelter waste, tailings and slag particles.
2. Ingesting or inhaling contaminated soils on site.
3. Ingesting or inhaling contaminated soil off site."

The report continued telling us that:

"Exposure to high levels of lead and arsenic can cause damages to blood cells, kidneys, and the gastrointestinal, reproductive and nervous systems. Both lead and arsenic are capable of crossing the placenta barrier and causing harm to the fetus of pregnant women. Evidence indicates that arsenic is a human carcinogen. Cadmium and certain forms of lead are classified as probable carcinogens, based on animal studies."

The ATSDR consultation determined that adult exposures did not exceed their Minimal Risk Levels but exposure to children living near the site exceeded the risk level standards. Conclusions in the health assessment stated that:

- "Although no biomonitoring data have been collected to provide information on actual exposure levels, the environmental levels of lead pose a likelihood that exposure has occurred and continues to occur for residents who live near the site and for visitors to the site.
- Arsenic, cadmium, and lead are the contaminants of concern, although lead is the contaminant present at levels that could cause adverse health effects, especially in children.
- Of particular concern is the potential for long term exposure developmental health effects on children residing near the site as a result of lead exposure.
- Although limited data indicates the surface water and groundwater are contaminated, off site migration of contaminants in the soil, surface water and groundwater may potentially extend to down gradient communities, thereby increasing the population potentially exposed."

ATSDR exposure reduction recommendations were:

- "Inform Lincoln residents supplied by individual wells of the potential for groundwater contamination and recommend testing for heavy metals.
- Improve access restrictions with effective measure such as replacing barbed wire fencing with more secure chain link fencing equipped with locked gates to keep trespassers off the site until final remediation is complete.
- Prevent further contamination of Dry Creek and Pine Creek with effective measures such as removing tailings and slag piles from drainage areas of both creeks and covering tailings and slag with soil caps.
- Establish erosion control measures to prevent contaminant migration off-site.
- Replace fallen, faded, or unreadable signs."

The report concluded with recommendations to be provided to the community. Health education would be provided to the exposed populations regarding the possible health effects from exposure site contaminants and about interim measures that can be taken to reduce exposures. Also, to provide free annual blood lead testing for children ages 6 months to 6 years of age living in the community of Lincoln.

Cleanup of the toxic site will take years and EPA funds are decreasing for such an extensive clean up. More information about toxic waste-site cleanup is contained in future chapters.

The ATSDR also sought information on other illnesses, such as Parkinson's disease and some respiratory ailments

Chronic Disease / Pollution Connection

that had been identified as community concerns. The report found that "currently insufficient data exists for descriptions or comparisons of these disease incidences at local, state, or nationals levels." This lack of data continues to hinder disease cluster studies and will be called to your attention in other studies.

The ATSDR was able to identify a disease cluster of lead poisoning in the Tooele area and to identify the cause since they had prevalence data and research for comparison. This is because lead poisoning is one of the few conditions tracked by many states. When you read about disease cluster health consultations performed by ATSDR, it is important to remember that they may be limited in what they can do if prevalence and disease research data is not available. Once again the need for a fully operational national disease tracking network is identified.

In 2001, the U.S. EPA reported that the state of Utah ranked fourth nationally in the release of toxic chemicals. In the 1950s and 1960s, tens of thousands of tons of radioactive materials were found there. Toxic waste is still being produced, brought to, and processed in Utah. In addition to what has been mentioned, there is a uranium mill in San Juan County where radioactive waste is recycled. Surprisingly, Utah continues to accept toxic waste. In other states, taxpayer money is being spent to clean up similar hazardous waste by moving it to places like Utah and creating another Superfund site (requiring EPA cleanup). We are running out of places to move toxic waste. Something is very wrong with this picture!

Chapter 5

Power Plants, Toxic Waste Incinerators and Nuclear Plants

Clusters of many diseases occur in areas surrounding power plants, toxic waste incinerators and nuclear plants. We will briefly look at each area.

Power Plants

Hundreds of coal-fired power plants are operating in the U.S. today. They are one of the top sources of mercury found in our air, water, and soil. Many plants operating today are between 30-50 years old and pollute our environment with ten times more nitrogen oxide and sulfur dioxide than modern power plants. In 1999, power plants polluted the air with 300,000 tons of fine carbon soot particles, which have been found to cause lung problems that contribute to lung disease and death.

Power plants are also causing major problems with pollution in state and national parks. The Great Smoky Mountains National Park in Tennessee has been reported to have the highest pollution levels in the national park system. Damage to trees, shrubs, and flowers has been reported. It is even difficult to view the beautiful mountains because of the ozone pollution. This is a common finding of visitors to the park area every year. It is not surprising to hear that Park Rangers are reporting respiratory problems.

The power in Great Smoky Mountains area is supplied by the Tennessee Valley Authority (TVA). The TVA burns coal to generate electricity and expels chemicals into the air. The TVA is said to be looking to improve methods for producing electrical power. The technology has been available for years, but it has not been generally utilized by coal burning power companies.

In 2002, the news media reported that the Sequoia National Forest had more ozone pollution than major cities in the U.S. Clean Air Act enforcement could control this problem, but is hindered by a loophole placed into the Act. Congress assumed that newer plants would soon replace the older, more polluting plants. This allowed many older coal-fired power plants to avoid modernizing with pollution controls. This loophole is allowed with little concern for the serious damage being done to the environment and to peoples' health.

Waste Incinerators

Toxic waste incinerators are suspected to be very harmful to people living in their shadows. Some of the most toxic substances are released by these incinerators. They are dioxin, furans, lead, and mercury. The suspected effects of exposure to these substances are damage to the nervous system, immune function, reproductive and developmental function, also kidney disease, liver diseases and cancers.

Chronic Disease / Pollution Connection

No State is unaffected by contamination from polluting industries. Even beautiful Vermont has problems. When we think of Vermont we think of ski slopes, green forests, and fresh air. In November, 2003 the Toxics Action Center in Montpelier released study results on toxic pollution in the state. The following results were reported for Vermont:

Active Hazardous Waste Sites:	1,360
Active Landfills:	2
Air Pollution Point Sources:	295
Closed/Inactive Landfill sites:	81
Fossil Fuel or Nuclear sites:	14
Large Quantity Hazardous Waste Generators:	116
Small Quantity Hazardous Waste Generators:	444
National Priority List (Superfund). Sites:	9
Water Discharges:	32
Pounds of Toxins Released in 2001:	363,002

This is just another example of the extent of the problems with pollution in America. Vermont suffers from the consequences of this pollution in damage to residents' health and to their once pristine environment. There are reports of neurological disease, birth defects, asthma, and cancer in the state. Clarendon, Vermont is now the location of a reported cancer disease cluster.

Health activists are starting to use the Clean Air Act and the Clean Water Act to force their states' EPA to take action against polluting industries in their neighborhoods. A citizen in southern Ohio used the Clean Air Act to successfully close down an industry that was polluting her neighborhood with extremely high levels of dioxin. It requires a great deal of determination, and persistence to be successful. Also you often have to be prepared to fight the industries' lawyers.

Nuclear Power Plants

Mysterious illnesses have been found for years surrounding nuclear plants and research centers and have been reportedly ignored by government agencies. Some insight into the health problems experienced by people living near nuclear facilities was detailed in the Nashville Tennessean newspaper. The newspaper published a series of articles in 1997 addressing problems found nationwide. The reports are titled "An Investigation into Illnesses Around the Nations Nuclear Weapons Sites. For the Ill, Help Is Often Out of Reach." The following information was found in the Tennessean:

> "A mysterious pattern of illnesses—from immune systems gone haywire to brain malfunctions that doctors can't explain—is emerging around the nation's nuclear weapons plants and research facilities.
>
> In 1997, the Tennessean found scores of people suffering a pattern of unexplained illnesses around the Oakridge nuclear reservation in East Tennessee. This year the newspaper found hundreds of people with similar illnesses around 10 other nuclear weapons sites nationwide."

One personal story was about a 41 year old man who described his condition as "like a devil has been let loose in my body." The newspaper provided the following information about this man:

> "The former worker at the U.S. Department of Energy's Savannah River nuclear site near Aiken, S.C. was declared disabled in 1995, suffering from a degenerative joint and spine disease, kidney ailments and a rare disorder that causes his immune system to

attack, rather than protect his internal organs. He is one of 410 people in 11 states interviewed by the Tennessean who are experiencing a pattern of unexplained immune, respiratory and neurological problems attacking their bodies and minds. The newspaper found ill residents and workers in Tennessee, Colorado, South Carolina, New Mexico, Idaho, New York, California, Ohio, Kentucky, Texas and Washington State."

The newspaper reports about cover ups and retaliations against whistle blowers and the harm done to individuals and the environment. For more information visit the newspaper's website www.tennessean.com. Or use your internet search engine to locate the story.

Dozens of studies have been performed at the Oakridge nuclear facility. You can review ATSDR reports at their website:

http://www.atsdr.cdc.gov/HAC/oakridge/phact/c_3.html.

Studies performed by the State of Tennessee reported no well documented studies that could be used for comparison at Oakridge. Thus again, it would be difficult, if not impossible, to make the chronic disease/pollution connection.

Chapter 6

Environmental Protection Agency (EPA)

The U.S.EPA was established in July of 1970 through the efforts of the White House and Congress, because of the growing public demand for cleaner water, air, and land. Its mission statement is to protect human health and to safeguard the natural environment. We should recognize that the U.S.EPA was given the task of cleaning up all the damage already done to the environment prior to July 1970. Some people question whether or not they have the power or funding to do their job.

It is important to understand the work the U.S.EPA does and their responsibilities to you. State EPA offices are set up in districts in every state, and their records can be viewed by the public. Efficiencies of state EPAs and their benefits to the public can vary from state to state.

My Experience With the EPA

The EPA is one of the first places to look to determine what is happening with polluting industries in your neighborhoods. When the foundry in Wellington, Ohio was shutting down, leaving an eight-acre waste dump site, a visit to the district OEPA office was very revealing. OEPA records clearly demonstrated what had transpired between the OEPA, the foundry, and the two other factories in the Wellington MS disease cluster area.

The plastics factory and the fertilizer company had some minor issues with the OEPA, but those had been resolved long ago. The Wellington foundry had stacks of correspondence in the OEPA files. The files provided detailed information on the company dating back from its origin in 1920. The records showed many years of non-compliance with OEPA standards. In one report, the foundry reported releases of chromium compounds, methanol, and phenol.

In November, 1995, a correspondence from the OEPA to the foundry addressed their failure to evaluate foundry waste. The foundry was directed to have samples analyzed for hazardous constituents and submit sampling results to the OEPA Northeast District Office. The foundry management did not comply. The district OEPA eventually referred the non-compliance to the managing OEPA office in Columbus, the state capital. The OEPA office eventually referred the problem to the Ohio State Attorney General. The state took the foundry to court in December 1998 for failure to meet EPA requirements and failure to clean up the eight-acre dump site.

I was able to access the actual docket records (Lorain County Common Pleas Court) on the web, using my computer. The only activities recorded for years were lawyers on both sides talking to each other by phone in "status conferences". Court dates had been set and changed repeatedly. The case had been in court 5 years the last time I checked public records, and remained unresolved at that time. The next scheduled legal review was set for spring 2005. Something is very wrong in our court system that allows this to happen. Meanwhile, the eight-acre foundry dump site remained exactly as it had been all those years.

The OEPA files also contained comments from staff saying, "It is questionable if samples were taken when a plant was in full operation." Testing of expelled products certainly would be affected by whether the furnaces, ventilating systems etc. were in full operation, partial operation, or closed down. The records revealed that testing at the foundry was not done by the OEPA, but by someone hired by the company to do the testing. This is typical, according to the staff, because the OEPA doesn't have funds to do their own testing. It is almost like the fox guarding the hen house; a pretty good analogy for this situation.

Staff at the District OEPA office was asked about their power to enforce relevant regulations. They reported that they cannot force a company to clean up their polluted site.

Chapter 7

Brownfields

The U.S.EPA is responsible for Brownfields in America. Brownfields are defined as abandoned or underused industrial and commercial facilities. New building construction on these Brownfield sites can cause community health problems when all contaminated soil and water are not cleaned up prior to new construction. The U.S. General Accounting Office estimates that there are 450,000 Brownfields across American. They are found in every state. Unfortunately, Brownfields are often given to communities and become the location of schools, housing, and parks.

The River Valley High School in Marion, Ohio

An example of a school built on a Brownfield and a chronic disease cluster occurred in Marion, Ohio. Marion is about 40 miles north of Columbus, the state capital. Marion had a leukemia problem that would pit citizen against citizen and government employee against government employee. It was a four-year battle that was widely covered by the media. Anyone interested can read a very detailed article by Hal Karp in the August 2000 Family Circle Magazine called "A

Town Divided: How a Cancer Threat is Tearing a Community Apart." The article provides more details about the personal experiences of the people living in Marion at that time.

The story of Marion involves a high school and a middle school built on a seventy eight acre campus that was once the site of two major military facilities operated by the Army. In 1993, a student at River Valley High School was diagnosed with a rare form of leukemia. In 1997, six other school graduates developed the same disease and soon the number reached eight victims. There were also cases of cancer of the esophagus and breast at the school. The school nurse contacted the state health department because of her concerns about the numbers. This resulted in a meeting between the county health officials, the ODH, and the OEPA. At the close of the meeting, they agreed that they needed to look into the problem.

At about the same time, parents of some of the cancer victims met and formed a group called Concerned River Valley Families (CRVF). Their purpose was to find out why their children were ill and how to stop the spread of the cancer. They immediately met opposition from other people in Marion, who felt the CRVF was ruining the reputation of the school and their town. The school board and a community development corporation also reportedly resented the publicity. This type of resentment can typically be found in most communities with disease clusters. The businesses fear it will affect their business, and city managers worry that the publicity will cause people to move from the community or not come to the community. People in the CRVF group reported harassment, threats, and one man said he was even shot at several times while mowing his lawn.

Chronic Disease / Pollution Connection

A Marion development corporation and the school board hired an environmental consulting firm to conduct testing at the school campus for any harmful substances. The firm they had hired conducted tests and concluded that there was no evidence of any contamination that would present a health hazard.

According to the Family Circle article:

> "At the same time, however, the OEPA began its own investigation and found evidence of 11 polycyclic aromatic hydrocarbons, chemical compounds formed when gasoline, garbage or other organic matters is burned. Six of the eleven were believed to be cancer producing. Topping the list was benzo(a)pyrene, which is thought to cause cancer when high levels are inhaled, ingested or absorbed through the skin. The amount found was forty times higher than the screening level, or levels of concern, set by the federal Environmental Protection Agency."

But, at that time, the OEPA reported that the school campus site posed no risk. So the students returned to the school that Fall as scheduled.

The OEPA later conducted further testing and found more contaminants, so the Army Corps of Engineers was called into the investigation. This was done because the site was a former defense site, which falls under the Army Corps of Engineers' jurisdiction. A report from the Army Corps of Engineers found no problems that were a threat to human health.

Then, a subcontractor hired by the Army Corps of Engineers contacted the U.S.EPA and the OEPA, saying that the study investigation was a fraud. He said he was told beforehand that he would not find any problems at the site. The U.S.EPA determined that the study in question was done correctly. The CRVF group refused to accept that conclusion.

The OEPA also had a whistleblower who said that the investigation was undermined by the OEPA from the beginning. He was fired from his position, but was reinstated after a federal judge ruled in his favor. The judge reprimanded the OEPA for limiting their investigation and knowingly and falsely finding that nothing in the environment was a threat to human health. The OEPA appealed the findings and asked for immunity. A later investigation relieved the OEPA of any wrong-doing.

Then the CRVF group, searching for information, found out about a safety director at the site's Scioto Ordinance Plant in the 1950s who had told of dumping toxic chemical waste, and of radioactive materials stored at a warehouse. This warehouse was located only a hundred yards from the River Valley School baseball field. This was after the Army Corps of Engineers assured people that there was not a problem there. The families also obtained an aerial photo, through public records at the Army's own archival research files, showing evidence of the dump site.

The Corps research showed twenty contaminants at River Valley Schools. The Corps did not dispute that chemicals at the subsurface level exceeded Primary Remedial Goal target levels set by the government. However, they contended that anyone playing or working at the surface level at River Valley Schools would not face a substantially increased risk of cancer, *as long as the surface soil layer was not broken.*

A Marion parent was quoted as saying that in certain portions of the subsurface, contaminated soil contained concentrations as high as 10% pure TCE at an 8-10 foot depth, which meant it was almost in the same state as it was when it was dumped 56 years earlier.

The Corps did not dispute the fact that chemicals are at the subsurface level and exceed the U.S. EPA target levels set by the government, but contended that anyone playing or working at the surface level of River Valley would not be at substantially increased risk of cancer.

The ODH began their study of the disease cluster in 1997. The study involved River Valley School graduates from 1963 to 2000. Unfortunately, the study was soon changed to look at leukemia cases in <u>all</u> of Marion County, and only from 1992 to 1999.

The ODH study results on July 26, 2000, came to three primary conclusions.

- "The most common factor among the leukemia victims was direct or secondhand tobacco smoke exposure.
- Sports or agricultural activities at the school could not be connected to six River Valley graduates' development of leukemia.
- Continued studies of leukemia among Marion County residents and River Valley graduates were unlikely to identify additional factors that caused the leukemia."

Marion residents scoffed at ODH findings, especially regarding cigarette smoking, saying there was no more smoking of cigarettes in their community than any other community.

Then Marion residents contacted a toxicologist working at the University of Pennsylvania to review the ODH report. The toxicologist was said to have found serious problems with the research results. For example, only 40% of the alumni responded to this survey. He felt that the ODH study treated the group as if it included the entire alumni population. He felt this made the number of leukemia cases far less significant. He also found that the ODH study showed that River Valley leukemia patients tended to be much younger than leukemia patients elsewhere in the county and they were much less likely to have smoked.

A later ODH study looking at cancer among River Valley graduates did find a higher than expected rate of esophageal cancer. However, no conclusions were drawn from the study, nor was any follow-up planned.

The students continued to attend classes at the schools until new schools were built elsewhere, funded in part by the U.S. Army Corps of Engineers. The new schools opened in Sept. 2003.

The U.S.EPA dug up tons of toxic creosote at the old school site. Creosote is an oily liquid with a pungent odor which is obtained from the distillation of coal tar. Exposure to creosote has been proven to cause severe skin irritation and kidney and liver damage. It is often used as a wood preservative. Some of this contaminated soil has been treated at the site and 3500 tons of soil were shipped to a hazardous landfill in Michigan. The U.S. EPA was said to be also considering dredging creosote from the Little Scioto River, a source for drinking water for Marion and for the state capital of Columbus.

Schools are built on Brownfields too often. If you question the safety of the land your child's school is built on, you can look up the information at your District EPA office.

Later you will read about the problems encountered when housing is built on a Brownfield.

Chapter 8

U.S.EPA Authority and Superfund Sites

Congress created Superfund in 1980 to require polluters to pay for cleanup. As time went by, the trust fund became more depleted and cleanups slowed dramatically. Most polluting industries closed down and filed for bankruptcy, leaving the cost of cleanup to be picked up by taxpayers through the U.S.EPA. A state's EPA can place a contaminated site on the National Priority List for cleanup, if the site is determined to be a threat to public health and meets all U.S.EPA criteria for cleanup.

Superfund sites are spread across America and should be of great concern to people everywhere. Reports tell us that one in four people live within four miles of a Superfund site, including ten million children. Also eighty five percent of Superfund sites have contaminated ground water. Fifty percent of U.S. citizens and one hundred percent of rural areas use ground water for drinking. Your county health department can provide testing for bacteria and nitrates, and some county laboratories are certified to perform other tests. Prices for water tests can vary widely.

You can find a laboratory in the yellow pages but always make sure to use a laboratory that has been certified to perform those particular tests.

I refer you again to the quick reference PIRG list, located in the appendix, for the most toxic chemicals found at Superfund sites and their adverse effects on health.

Chronic disease clusters frequently occur at Superfund sites; in fact most Superfund sites have multiple disease clusters.

Massachusetts Disease Clusters.

An example of a multiple disease cluster located in close proximity to a Superfund site was occurring at the time of this writing in 2004. Four Massachusetts communities, Abington, Weymouth, Rockland, and Middleboro, had chronic disease clusters and were undergoing public health investigations. The controversy involves the South Weymouth US Naval Air Station, its jet fuel pipeline running under nearby communities, and its toxic Superfund site located in close proximity to the disease clusters.

These public health investigations resulted from pressure by community health advocates in the area. And this was largely because of efforts by their very active MS support group named Abington, Weymouth, And Rockland Environmental Studies (AWARES). This group has worked very hard to find reasons for so many ill people in the area.

Liz is one of the health activist involved in the support group. Liz, who has MS, decided to do her own study when she saw that state and federal investigations would take years, while people were continuing to be diagnosed with chronic diseases. She believed help was needed more quickly, and initiated a very large survey of people throughout the area using a detailed questionnaire that she developed. The survey looked at all chronic diseases and was intended to reach every home. Liz felt that was the only way to convince public health care agencies that there are many more ill people than the agencies believed, and that people were continuing to get newly diagnosed with serious diseases. Completing the health study would provide better numbers and locations of the diseases in the area surrounding the Naval Base. Liz's survey was very labor intensive and has required months of work, and was still in process at the time of this writing. If there had been a fully operational chronic disease tracking network, health officials could have quickly determined the numbers and locations of cases. Then the spread of disease could have been investigated more quickly, rather than waiting years while people continued to get sick. Since that was not the case, health advocates like Liz placed their lives on hold while searching for answers in hopes of stopping the spread of diseases in their communities.

Liz was just beginning to look at the survey numbers. She reported that she had already found sixty cases of MS in close proximity of the air base, and also cases of Amyotrophic Lateral Sclerosis (ALS) (also known as Lou Gehrig's disease), lupus, Parkinson's disease, asthma, and autism. ALS is a devastating terminal disease that affects nerve conduction to muscles throughout the body. This causes progressive paralysis, first usually in extremities, and then in muscles involved in respiration, eventually causing death in two to five years. Parkinson's is a debilitating degenerative neuromuscular disease. Lupus is a chronic inflammatory disease causing abnormalities in blood vessels and connective tissue. The causes of these diseases are not known, but scientists are looking more and more at toxic environmental exposure.

The South Weymouth Naval Air Station closed in 1997 leaving a toxic Superfund site. The site was being purchased by a group planning to put in housing, recreation facilities, and shopping areas. The Navy wanted to transfer the area and let construction begin. The AWARE group had focused on stopping transfer of the land because they were concerned that people would quickly move into the area and could then become exposed to chemicals seeping from the base area. The AWARE group was successful in having land transfer to the development corporation postponed until June 2004. Liz was relieved, and reported that "The EPA has not even done a water assessment. They don't even know what is running off the base into nearby wells and streams and backyards". <u>In May, 2004 the transfer of property to the development corporation proceeded despite what the support group was promised.</u>

Massachusetts State officials have completed a cancer study that found elevated levels of lung cancer in the area. They found no definitive cause, but cigarette smoking was suggested. A two-year study of this disease cluster area by the Massachusetts State Department of Health was reported to be started soon.

A separate State investigation was being conducted to determine the source of arsenic contamination involving six South Weymouth families. There was another study being conducted by state health officials in Middleboro, where twenty-seven individuals have been diagnosed with ALS. They reportedly lived within a one-mile radius of a hazardous waste site. State health studies in Abington, Weymouth, and Rockland were expected to be completed in 2005.

Chapter 9

Heavy Metal Poisoning in the U.S

Heavy metals are linked to human poisoning and cause serious nervous system damage, cancers, and problems with growth and development. Some metals such as lead are reported to cross the placenta and cause fetal brain damage. Other metals are reported to attack the immune system causing autoimmune diseases and also diseases of the kidneys and circulatory system. Sources of heavy metal pollution include waste from metal mining and metal industries, and air emissions from coal burning plants, smelters, and waste incinerators.

Certain types of industrial facilities are required to report their heavy metal releases to the EPA Toxic Release Inventory. <u>Unfortunately, some major industries like waste incinerators are not required to report.</u> Consequently, the Toxic Release Inventory may significantly under-estimate environmental releases of some metals. Heavy metal releases are reported to remain in the environment for decades or centuries.

We will look at two very toxic heavy metals found in our environment. They are lead covered in this chapter, and mercury in the following chapter. Both cause very serious public health damage.

Lead Contamination

Lead poisoning continues to be a problem even though lead based paint was banned in 1978 because of its proven very toxic effects. Yet here are some places where lead can still be found today according to the U.S. EPA.

- "Lead is still found inside and outside homes in old lead-based paint.
- Lead is found in soil around homes because soil can hold lead from past use of leaded gasoline in cars and other gasoline powered vehicles and machinery.
- Hobbies that use lead are also a problem in the home when making pottery, stained glass or refinishing furniture.
- Lead in homes can come from plumbing with lead pipes or with lead solder on pipes."

You can not see, smell, or taste lead in water, and boiling water will not get rid of lead. Many communities are using leaded pipe lines to this day. The U.S.EPA recommends that you call your local health departments to find out about testing your water, if you have concerns about leaded water pipes contaminating your water.

Other U.S.EPA identified sources of lead are old painted toys and furniture, and food stored in lead crystal. Yes, ladies, those beautiful leaded crystal glasses leech lead into the wine, water, and other beverages. Crystal manufacturers are said to be voluntarily reducing the amount of lead in lead crystal even though a great deal of 24% lead crystal is still being sold in virtually all department stores across America.

The U.S.EPA recommendations for the use of lead crystal are as follows:

- "Do not use lead crystal everyday.
- Do not store liquids in lead crystal glasses, bottles, or dishes.
- Do not allow alcoholic beverages to sit in your crystal glass for long periods of time.
- Do not feed children from lead crystal containers."

Children exposed to high levels of lead can suffer from damage to the brain and nervous system. They may also have behavior and learning problems, slowed growth and development, hearing problems, and headaches. Adults can suffer from difficulties during pregnancy and have reproductive problems, high blood pressure, digestive problems, nerve disorders, memory and concentration problems, and muscle and joint pain.

The Department of Health and Human Services has determined that lead acetate and lead phosphate may reasonably be anticipated to cause cancer. This is based on animal studies but it has not been proven in people. You will find this explanation regarding many chemical exposure studies that stop short of identifying the toxic source of the human cancer or other chronic diseases because of lack of scientific proof.

Stories from some communities provide some insight into the impact of lead on the environment and public health today.

Roseville and Crooksville, Ohio

Roseville and Crooksville, in the southeastern part of Ohio, were once home to the pottery industry. The potteries used lead glazes on their pottery and heavy lead contamination was suspected in old pottery dump sites. Contaminated soil was found throughout Roseville and Crooksville, including residential soil, community parks, ball fields, and school property. The history of residents using discarded pottery waste on their roads and sidewalks probably contributed to the extent of the contamination. The safe standard for lead in soil at an industrial site is 1800 part per million (ppm). In a residential site, 400 ppm is considered safe. The OEPA study found lead levels higher than 5,000 ppm at five former pottery sites in Roseville and at one pottery site in nearby Crooksville. Each site had levels of 11,000 ppm in some samples. Two sites, the Roseville Elementary School parking lot and a former pottery disposal site, both had levels of 80,500 ppm. The US EPA recommended removing and replacing contaminated soil and erecting permanent barriers around properties with levels of lead higher than 5000 ppm. The big problem is that the pottery companies had closed years ago. No one seemed to know who will pay to clean up this lead contamination. Two site cleanups were initiated around the Rosewood Elementary School and a trailer park. Roseville officials continued to look for funding to clean up their community.

In November 1997, the Ohio EPA and the ODH were to meet with the community, and the ODH was to offer blood screenings for lead toxicity. The EPA recommended the protection of children from the high concentrations of lead found in the soil. The ODH instructed residents on measures to protect children. On April 14, 2005, the ODH provided a one day training course to individuals and construction companies on safe lead renovation.

Pottery production in the U.S. is said to now use low-lead and no-lead glazes and presents no problems. However, the

Chronic Disease / Pollution Connection |

U.S. EPA warns that imported ceramics and pottery often still have lead glazes. I know you will be checking the bottom of your dishes just as I did.

Eastern Shores of Virginia, Accomack County

A high rate of lead poisoning was found in the Eastern Shores county of Accomack, Virginia. In an eighteen month period in 2003, eighty six children under age six were diagnosed with lead poisoning. The Accomack-Hampton Planning District Commission was awarded a grant to reduce lead hazards in sixty low-income housing units, which had been constructed before lead paint was banned for residential use. The state implemented the Virginia Lead Safe Home Program to educate people throughout the state about the dangers of lead poisoning.

Picher, Oklahoma's Unique Solution

More than 30 years after mining operations ended, dozens of mounds of lead-contaminated gravel and sand remain in Tar Creek, near Picher, Oklahoma, population 1,640. The mining company reportedly left seventy five million tons of contaminated waste in and around Picher.

The EPA has known about the contamination and is reported to have struggled over the years to protect residents in the area that became known as Americas #1 Superfund Site. Dust clouds from the waste piles spread lead, cadmium, and other pollutants throughout the community. Outside the town, acidic water from abandoned mines has poisoned streams and colored the woods a bright orange color. Nearby mine shafts, hundreds of feet deep, are open and unprotected by fences. Pictures of the area make you think you are seeing a horror movie or a scene found in an end of the world scenario.

In the Picher area, the number of children under six years of age with elevated levels of lead in their blood was 11.9% in the year 2000. The national average is 1.9%. Community members say that the public health estimates grossly underestimated the number of poisoned children, because only one child was tested in each of the randomly selected homes.

Land next to a school was found to contain lead contamination forty times higher than acceptable levels. School officials reported that more than half of a select group of twenty eight pupils with high lead levels are having learning problems.

Local critics felt that the EPA spent millions of dollars cleaning leaded soil from hundreds of backyards without doing anything about the source of the contamination.

The State of Oklahoma is now asking the federal government for $250 million dollars to move the towns. This sounds like a radical solution for solving an environmental pollution problem. Still, millions of dollars have been spent to clean up the lead contamination and the problem remains. Picher and close-by Cardin, population 200, would be reestablished elsewhere with new homes, streets, and new schools. The hope would be to convert the toxic swath of land in Oklahoma into a 2500 acre wetland and reservoir. You may remember a similar situation when people were moved from Love Canal in the state of New York, where homes had been built on top of a toxic dump site.

Treatment for Lead Poisoning

As mentioned earlier, children are most susceptible to lead contamination and have the most damage. Physicians can treat children having very high levels of lead in their bodies. Treatment includes vitamin therapy, diets rich in iron and calcium, and Chelation Therapy. Chelation Therapy uses medication to remove lead from the blood. The problem is that the children are being found too late, after the damage has already been done. Some pediatricians report that they are ordering lead screening on all children suspected of living in potentially contaminated low income housing where leaded paint can still be found. Reports of lead poisoning are found in almost every state in the U.S. Some states are requiring lead blood level testing on all children entering kindergarten.

Adult treatment for lead poisoning is similar to that of children. Adults require more Chelation Therapy, depending on the lead levels in their blood.

Lead Problems Continue

Lead poisoning in the environment remains a big problem in this country from more than old lead contaminated sites. Lead smelting industries, as well as other industries, continue to be major sources of lead pollution because they release lead into our air, water, and land on a daily basis.

In early July 2004, the news media announced the largest toy recall in U.S. history and warned people about children's jewelry sold in vending machines across the country. The jewelry contained toxic levels of lead. So even though the dangers of lead poisoning have been known for years, you have no choice but to arm yourself with the information needed to protect yourself and your family. Some times you cannot tell where an item is made and what the contents are in a product, but thankfully that is becoming less of a problem.

Chapter 10

Mercury Contamination

Another of the most toxic substances found in our environment is mercury. Coal-fired power plants are the countries largest unregulated source of mercury pollution. The National Institute of Health reports that:

> "The nervous system is very sensitive to all forms of mercury. Methyl mercury and metallic mercury vapors are more harmful than other forms, because more mercury in these forms reaches the brain. Exposure to high levels of metallic, inorganic, or organic mercury can permanently damage the brain, kidneys, and developing fetuses."

Some studies have shown that one in six U.S. women of childbearing age have mercury blood levels high enough to harm a developing fetus. In children, mercury causes learning problems and brain damage.

The ATSDR reports that we can be exposed to mercury in the following ways:

- "Eating fish and shellfish contaminated with methylmercury.

- Breathing vapors in the air, from incinerators and industries that burn mercury-containing fuels.
- Through contaminated workplace air or skin contact during use in the workplace (dental, health services, chemical, and other industries that use mercury).
- Releases from dental work and medical treatments."

In May 2005, an environmental support group was offering screenings for mercury to the public for a twenty five dollar fee. Maybe this venture will provide us with more information on the extent of damage done by mercury exposure.

Hoboken, New Jersey Mercury Contamination

The story of mercury contamination in Hoboken, New Jersey clearly points to the harm that can be done to the unsuspecting public. In Hoboken, mercury found its way into the environment in an unusual way. It points out the problems found when construction on an old industrial site (Brownfield) was rushed to completion before the site has been cleaned up. This practice happens all too often in this country. The happening in Hoboken, New Jersey is a prime example of what can go wrong.

An EPA website contained a report entitled "Army Corps of Engineers Assists EPA in New Jersey Superfund Cleanup". The report explained that a Hoboken resident was working in her apartment kitchen when she found a substance dripping from the ceiling onto her countertop. Health officials were called to investigate and discovered mercury underneath the five story apartment building's wooden floorboards that had absorbed into the walls. Mercury is a silvery white metallic element that is poisonous to humans and is the only metal that exists as a liquid at room temperature. Investigators also detected mercury vapor in the air, which can be toxic when inhaled.

From 1910 to 1965, the building had been the location of a General Electric plant that produced mercury vapor lamps and mercury connector switches. Mercury vapor lamps were used as street lamps and were popular in the early part of the 20th century. In the early to mid-1990s the building was converted into art studios and sixteen residential apartments.

The U.S.EPA investigated the building and decided that it needed to be cleaned up as soon as possible. The 27,000 square-foot apartment building with an attached four story brick town house was quickly closed. General Electric was required under administrative order to pay for the cleanup. The EPA asked the Army Corps of Engineers to supervise the cleanup. The Corps also assisted the EPA in evacuating and relocating sixteen families and twenty businesses that had occupied the area.

The cleanup involved demolishing the buildings and removing and disposing of the contaminated soil and other materials off site. Workers disassembled buildings by hand and demolishing brick walls using jackhammers. The floors were removed one bay at a time and inspected for mercury. Concrete slabs and subsurface piping were removed. Mercury contamination was removed from the surrounding soil. During cleanup, measures were said to be taken to protect the surrounding neighborhood communities by management facilities in New Jersey and Pennsylvania. Debris contaminated with mercury was shipped to hazardous waste landfills in New York and

Alabama. Liquid mercury was recycled. The non-hazardous solid waste and asbestos containing materials removed during cleanup were sent to specially designated waste sites.

Approximately 40,000 residents lived within a one-mile radius of this site. A high school and a residential community were also closed because of the threat to public health. The EPA found unsafe levels of mercury throughout the Hoboken site. Mercury levels in the air were 1,000 times safe levels. Residents were referred to a clinic that specializes in environmental health problems where they would be monitored for toxic symptoms.

When mercury blood levels are very high, Chelation Therapy is used for treatment. This is the same treatment used for lead poisoning mentioned earlier.

Chapter 11

Cancer and the Environmental Connection

There is a great deal of information available regarding cancer in the United States. A CDC report titled "Preventing and Controlling Cancer: Addressing the Nation's Second Leading Cause of Death" reported that:

"In 2002 cancer was the second leading cause of death for Americans and was responsible for one in four deaths. About sixteen million new cancer cases were diagnosed between 1990 and 2002. These estimates did not include in situ (preinvasive) cancer or the cases of nonmelanoma skin cancers.

Black Americans are more likely to die from cancer than people of any other racial or ethnic group. From 1992 to 1998, the average annual death rate per 100,000 people for all cancers combined was 218.2 for blacks, 164.5 for whites, 105.4 for American Indians/Alaska Natives, 102.6 for Hispanics, and 101.2 for Asians/Pacific Islanders."

The financial costs of cancer are staggering. According to the National Institute of Health (NIH), in 2004 the direct costs of cancer care in the United States totaled $189.8 billion.

There is high risk of cancer in communities located near polluting industries and toxic sites for adults as well as children. Cancer studies involving toxic waste sites have found increased adult deaths from breast, lung, and bladder cancer, and also cancer of the esophagus, stomach, large intestines, and rectum. Researchers believe that there may be as many as 100 kinds of cancer and they may have a latency period before symptoms appear. This makes it even more difficult to pin-point a cause. Some researchers believe that most cancers are likely caused by a combination of heredity and environmental factors. Environmental factors could include air, water, soil in the area, diet, and the use of tobacco, alcohol, and drugs. Exposures can occur inside the home or in the workplace. It can also include exposure to chemicals, sunlight, and other forms of radiation. Hereditary cancer is believed to develop because of genetic mutation that can be passed on to generation after generation. If you have an inherited risk factor, it does not mean that cancer will occur unless other factors created in the environment occur and promote cancer growth.

Research using animal studies has found a direct connection between toxic exposure and the development of cancer. More research needs to be done on the effects of toxic exposure for humans. Air releases of the metals cadmium, nickel, and chromium are believed to cause lung cancer. Vinyl chloride can cause liver cancer. Exposure to arsenic is suspected to cause skin and lung cancer. Leukemia is suspected to be caused from exposure to benzene and cyclophosphamide which cause changes in bone marrow. It seems reasonable for scientific research to focus on causes and cures for cancer in humans and less on treatments, but that is not the case for most research.

National Cancer Registry

A program meant to closely monitor cancer in the United State is the National Program of Cancer Registry. The CDC's National Program of Cancer Registry was authorized by Congress in 1992 and is defined as a systematic collection and analysis of cancer data. The information is critical for directing effective cancer prevention and control programs. Physicians are expected to report all newly diagnosed cancer cases to their state health departments. Statewide cancer registries help identify and monitor trends in cancer incidence and mortality, and guides cancer control planning and evaluation. They also help to allocate health funds, and advance clinical, epidemiologic, and health research. In short, a great deal depends on accurate information from the states.

Trust For Americas Health (TFAH) has investigated and evaluated each state's Cancer Registry with a grading system. TFAH is a nonprofit public health advocacy organization taking action to prevent diseases and protect the health and safety of our communities. TFAH's stated objectives are "to advocate for health policies that protect our communities health, develop tools to effectively tackle today's health problems, and give everyone the information they need to fight disease." You can find your state's grade in a June 2003 report titled "How Well Are States Tracking Cancer."

In the TFAH report you will find the following information:

> "California, Colorado, Idaho, and Illinois received an A grade for management of their cancer disease registry. Most states did get a good grade, but Maine, North Dakota and Tennessee received a D grade. Mississippi received the only F grade. Sixteen states including Ohio are listed as NA."

The NA means that the state health department did not send the requested information; therefore their cancer registry could not be evaluated. Consequently, any health department using the Cancer Registry to count cancer cases in a disease cluster study could have varying degrees of accuracy depending on the particular state's management of their Registry.

Nez Perce County, Idaho

An example of an adult cancer disease cluster was found in Nez Perce County, Idaho, which was home to pulp and paper mills established in 1952. The mills are located on 787 acres northeast of Lewiston, Idaho. Approximately 16,000 people live within a 3 mile radius of the facility.

The wood pulp made in the paper production is bleached in a process that releases chloroform into the air, and chloroform is a known carcinogen. Cancers associated with chloroform exposure are lung, kidney and bladder, rectal, prostate, and liver.

The community surrounding the industry reported elevated rates of many types of cancer and the ATSDR agreed to perform a health consultation. The ATSDR reported significantly more colon cancer, female kidney and pelvis cancer, as well as elevated numbers of rectal, lung, and prostate cancer in the Nez Perce area. The report from the ATSDR consultation was published in Sept.2003 and came to the following conclusions:

- "Chloroform concentrations measured in both indoor and outdoor air in residential areas are unlikely to cause any adverse non-carcinogenic public health effects considering air releases after 1992.
- Based on Chloroform concentrations in the downwind sampling location in 1990, theoretically, the estimated cancer risk is about 40 times higher than

that exposure to the national background chloroform. No data is available for BEHS to evaluate exposure prior to 1990.
- Health outcome data analysis indicates more cancer (12%) than expected for this area compared to the remainder of Idaho. Currently, it is not possible for BEHS to determine if past exposure to site related chloroform is associated with the increased incidence."

The BEHS mentioned refers to the Bureau of Environmental Health and Safety. The BEHS is responsible for providing the citizens with a high level of health protection. The bureau apparently lacked the past exposure information needed in the Nez Perce study as evidenced by the study conclusions. Once again environmental health studies performed by the government concluded that no earlier data was available for a comparison, so results of a disease cluster study are inconclusive or can not make a chronic disease / pollution connection. The ATSDR suggested cigarette smoking and diets high in fat and low in fiber could have contributed of these cancers in Nez Perce.

The ATSDR recommendations for residents were:

- "Residents should use kitchen and bathroom exhaust fans when cooking and showering, and should maintain good ventilation in the home to minimize chloroform accumulation from water use, since indoor air chloroform concentrations are higher than outdoor concentrations.
- Cancer surveillance in the community should continue."

The ATSDR also performed a health consultation in Nez Perce to assess possible health risk to the community from benzene exposure. Benzene levels were elevated in the area, but their studies concluded that benzene was not likely to be the source of the cancer. However, as shown in appendix C, Benzene is a known source of cancer causing chemicals.

Then I found two separate events that provide more information on the Nez Perce County's problems. In April 2003, an Idaho environmental support group challenged the air quality model used by the mill for monitoring air pollution. This was due to the fact that the air quality model used by the mill was not capable of accounting for the placement of a mill at the bottom of a 2000 foot canyon. The valley surrounding the mill was found to create a hydrogen sulfide cold air cap over the area causing the pollution levels to increase at night.

The second more surprising event was an EPA Notice of Lodging a Consent Decree Under Clean Air Act against the paper mill in November 1998. This is "a legal document, approved by a judge, which formalizes an agreement reached between the EPA and Potentially Responsible Parties. The Potentially Responsible Party agrees to conduct all or part of a cleanup action at a Superfund site, and to cease or correct actions or processes that are polluting the environment." According to the decree, the claims were said to have been in connection to the asbestos removal activities performed during the renovation/demolition at the mill in 1992. In other words, the mill may have seriously contaminated the area with asbestos.

The company was required to pay a penalty of $30,000 for their actions. The company was also instructed to follow EPA standards when working with asbestos, and to provide training for their personnel. The company was also required to report their activities monthly to the US EPA.

I have two comments about the information above.

- A penalty of $30,000 isn't much of a penalty for a large corporation to pay for polluting the county and exposing people to asbestos.
- I was not able to find any asbestos health problems being addressed by the U.S.EPA, the Utah Health Department, or the ATSDR in Nez Perce County. Asbestos exposure has been proven to cause cancer of the lungs, digestive tract, colon, larynx, esophagus, kidney, and some types of lymphoma. That doesn't mean that the problem was totally missed but I was unable to confirm any public health agency involvement regarding asbestos exposure.

In 2003, the Cancer Registry reported elevated cancer rates in Nez Perce County, as did the heath consultation by the ATSDR, so this is reason for concern. You will understand my concern when you learn more about the serious health problems caused by asbestos exposure.

It may be surprising to some people to hear about continuing health damage from asbestos exposure, since the danger has been known for many years. The information on asbestos contamination in the following chapter should paint a clear picture about the continuing serious problems.

Chapter 12

Asbestos and Silica Exposure Problems

The continuing asbestos damage to Americans' health is alarming healthcare providers across the country. People continue to be diagnosed with asbestos related diseases. Such diseases are now known to have up to a forty year latency period, the time from exposure to the beginning of symptoms.

Libby, Montana Asbestos Manufacturing Site

Asbestos fibers were contained in Zololite home insulation used in homes across the United States from about 1930 to 1980. People were unaware that Zololite contained asbestos fiber. The insulation was produced at large vermiculite ore mines in Libby, Montana, a town of 2600 people where at least 200 miners, family members, and residents died from exposure to asbestos fibers.

The Libby mines closed in 1990, and about 10 years later the mining company filed for bankruptcy. Then, in February, 2005 the United States Department of Justice and the

U.S.EPA announced a federal grand jury indictment against the manufacturer. The indictment stated that the manufacturer and its executives, as far back as 1970's, attempted to hide the fact that toxic asbestos was present in vermiculite products. The grand jury charged the company with conspiring to conceal information about the hazardous nature of the company's products, obstructing a government cleanup effort, and wire fraud. According to the indictment, 1200 residents of Libby have been identified as suffering from some kind of asbestos related disease. No further information about the results of the indictment was available at the time of this book's writing. The company categorically denied any wrong doing.

Relevant information about asbestos and asbestos related diseases can be found in a June 20, 2002 presentation by Gregory R. Wagner, M.D. He is Director, Division of Respiratory Disease Studies, The National Institute for Occupational Safety and Health at the CDC. The information was presented to the Senate Subcommittee on Environment and Public Works. Some highlights include the following information:

"Regulatory action and liability concerns related to the now well-established connection between inhalation of asbestos fibers and a variety of serious and often fatal diseases have reduced or eliminated the use of asbestos in many commercial products. However, asbestos and asbestos-containing materials are still found in many residential and commercial settings and pose a risk of exposure to workers and others.

Exposure to asbestos significantly increases the risk of contracting several diseases. These include:

1. Asbestosis—a disease characterized by scarring of the air-exchange regions of the lungs;
2. Lung cancer—for which asbestos is one of the leading causes among nonsmokers, and which occurs at dramatically high rates among asbestos-exposed smokers;
3. Malignant mesothelioma—an almost invariably fatal cancer of the tissue lining the chest or abdomen for which asbestos and similar fibers are the only known cause; and
4. Nonmalignant pleural disease—which can appear as a painful accumulation of bloody fluid surrounding the lungs, but which more commonly is seen as thick and sometimes constricting scarring of the tissue surrounding the lungs.

In addition, asbestos exposure is associated with excess mortality due to cancer of the larynx and cancer of the gastrointestinal tract. The malignant diseases—the cancers including mesothelioma—are often fatal within a year or a few years of initial diagnosis. In contrast, asbestosis deaths typically occur only after many years of suffering from impaired breathing".

Asbestos diseases can occur in family members when they come in contact with asbestos dust or fibers brought into the home on clothing, hair, or skin of the asbestos workers.

A few places today where people are still exposed to asbestos are in the construction trades and auto repair. The exposure occurs to construction workers through insulation covering on pipes, boilers and industrial furnaces. Auto repair exposure occurs when mechanics work with brakes and transmission products.

The Libby, Montana area has been the focus of a number of health studies. In December 2000 the ATSDR published the following health consultation results:

- "48 % (159 of 328) of the former manufacturer employees who participated in the medical testing had pleural abnormalities (pleural refers to the lining of the chest cavity that contains the lungs).
- Most reported multiple routes of exposure to asbestos contaminated vermiculite; 24% of the participants reported six or more routes of exposure (household, occupational, recreational, etc) had pleural abnormalities.
- 5% of those who participated reported no apparent exposure but had pleural abnormalities."

The ATSDR staff also reviewed death certificate data from 1979 to 1998 in the Libby community. The review found that the deaths from asbestosis in the Libby area were at least 40 to 60 times higher than expected. They also found that mesothelioma numbers appeared to be elevated. In 2002 the ATSDR was working to transfer medical testing and transition follow up to state and local health departments.

Another ATSDR report on Sept.9, 2003 focuses on the difficulties involved in studying asbestos exposure. In the ATSDR report titled, "National Asbestos Exposure Review", they released the following information on Libby to the public:

"Evaluating the health effects of exposure to Libby asbestos requires extensive knowledge of both exposure pathways and toxicity data. The toxicological information currently available is limited, and therefore the exact level of health concern for different sizes and types of asbestos remains controversial.

- Site-specific exposure pathway information is also limited or unavailable. There is limited information on past concentrations of Libby asbestos in air and around the plant.
- Significant uncertainties and conflicts in the methods used to analyze asbestos exist. These limitations make it hard to estimate the levels of Libby asbestos that people may have been exposed to.
- There is not enough information known about how and how often people came in contact with the Libby asbestos from the plant, because most exposures happened so long ago. This information is necessary to estimate accurate exposure doses.
- There is not enough information available about how some vermiculite materials, such as waste rock, were handled or disposed. This lack of information makes it difficult to identify and assess potential current exposures.
- Given these difficulties, the public health implications of past operations at this site can be evaluated only qualitatively."

This lack of data must have been extremely frustrating to the ATSDR members conducting studies in Libby. The ATSDR has also been given the task of accessing about 200 communities where Libby asbestos was sent.

Minnesota Congressman Bruce Vento also became a victim of asbestos exposure. He was exposed to asbestos during a three month period when he worked at a summer job as a college student. He died of Mesothelioma in 2000, thirty five years later. Media reported that, weeks before his death he filed eleven lawsuits against companies that allegedly supplied or installed asbestos products at the job sites where he had worked as a state paid laborer. He left behind a wife and three sons.

Even in 2005, the medical community and public health agencies had great concerns about what has happened in Libby. This was evidenced by many media reports and government communications regarding asbestos-related health problems. Many people continued to suffer from asbestos exposure, and help often reaches these people too late. This is just another obvious example of how an efficient, fully operational U.S. disease tracking network would have saved lives. It would have sent up a red flag years ago about what was happening in Libby. The high incidence of diseases among workers and their families could have focused a search for finding a common exposure.

Do we need to worry about asbestos exposure today? Yes, we do have to worry. Many asbestos products are still in use today, posing serious exposure risks when they are handled, repaired, or damaged. Old toasters and irons should be handled carefully because asbestos is found in old appliances and in their wiring. Recent media reports tell of the problems involved in removal of asbestos insulation found in some public schools and other older buildings in cities across America. People must be proactive in protecting themselves and their families. If you are unsure about asbestos in a school, residential building, or factory, ask questions and get answers. Asbestos exposure consequences remain a huge problem and, with the extended latency period involved, the problems could be with us for many years to come.

Silicosis

Silicosis is another disease whose cause has been known for years and yet it continues to harm people. Silica dust is from an inorganic compound, silicon dioxide. It is found in sands, quartzes, flints and many stones. Occupations at risk for silicosis include workers involved in mines, foundries, blasting operations, stone, glass, and clay manufacturing, and sandblasting. Also included are any operations involving working with rocks (crushing, loading, chipping, etc.)

Silicosis is a disease caused by exposure to free crystalline silica dust. This causes fibroid nodules in lungs. Patients with silicosis can have shortness of breath, weight loss, and persistent cough. These individuals are also at high risk for developing rheumatoid arthritis, autoimmune diseases, heart failure, and other lung diseases such as cancer, tuberculosis, bronchitis, and emphysema. Each person's disease process can vary depending on the length of exposure and concentrations of free silica dust in their work environment. There is no known cure for silicosis, and treatment focuses on slowing the progression of the disease and treating complications with drugs.

I would like to share a very informative speech regarding silicosis and exposure to silica dust. The presentation was made by Frances Perkins, U.S. Secretary of Labor, at a U.S. Government Conference in Joplin Missouri on April 23, 1940. <u>Yes, I said 1940.</u> She stated the following profound words:

"In the past 25 years we have become conscious of silicosis, not only in mines and tunnels and open cut foundations, but also in factories and mills where people work upon a substance which generate a silica dust or have silica bases. So having become conscious of this disease and its extent, it is our duty in the US Department of Labor of the United States to see if we can find ways to prevent it.

This morning I spoke with a group of women here in the mining area. They told me in their own simple words, that they and their children and their husbands, many of them, had what they regard as of the lung disease. Some of them spoke with bitterness and some with questions and some with resignation. There was only one thing I could say for slight comfort to these women who have lost their husbands or whose little children are infected. It was that by cooperating with the doctor, and the county health nurse, the State Medical Society, and the State Tuberculosis Society, perhaps they could make it possible not only for their own children to be cured, but for others whom they did not know, who are perhaps yet to be born, to be protected from the ravages of this disease.

So I say to you that although some of you may not like the idea of this Tristate area being used as a laboratory, can you not think of it is perhaps a great privilege? You may work out the methods by which thousands of others, millions of others, perhaps yet unborn may be protected from the hazards, which I know you employers, taxpayers, labor people regret as much as we in the Department of Labor do. Perhaps by the use of this as a laboratory you may contribute more to the welfare of this community and the whole United States, than anyone has yet thought.

All of us here today have a social responsibility, a moral responsibility, and perhaps the lesser degree of responsibility, which I will call legal responsibility. For the latter is not as important as a social and moral responsibility.

The owners and operators of these properties have a great moral responsibility, and many of them have acknowledged it. That is one of the things that gives us courage to come here and asked them to cooperate in making a laboratory in their area, to find a way to prevent not only this but similar situations everywhere.

The people who work in those mines and those who represent organized labor of the community generally also have a moral responsibility to cooperate with every technical and economic effort to relieve the situation and to find the means of preventing silicosis and tuberculosis."

The speech began with the statement that employee health problems had been recognized in mining industries for 25 years. So we are talking about problems found in **1915**. We can only imagine how many more people would have been spared the suffering of serious health problems and could have lived a full life if the government and the mining industry had acted at that time.

In the past, silicosis typically occurred in elderly populations, usually following many years of silica dust exposure. Silicosis deaths today, however, are occurring in younger populations, usually following recent overexposure. More than one million U.S. workers are exposed to crystalline silica. To this day, people are continuing to be harmed by exposure to silica dust because laws and regulations are not being enforced. The disease is preventable if employers would follow required protective measures. These measures include supplying workers with respirators and periodic health exams. Workers may not be aware of the dangers and they may not know what protective measures should be adhered to when working around silica dust.

Chapter 13

Childhood Disease Clusters–Asthma

Toxic chemicals in the environment have a greater impact on children for a number of reasons. Their immune systems, respiratory systems, and nervous systems are immature and develop at a rapid rate. Children are not able to detoxify and excrete toxic chemicals as well as adults. In early years they spend time playing on floors and in yards and typically put everything in their mouth. Even though science has recognized the toxic effects of some chemicals like lead on children, knowledge is lacking regarding the effects of many other chemicals. Long-term low-level chemical exposure effects have only recently begun to be explored.

Childhood disease clusters are occurring across America. These disease clusters include asthma, cancer, and birth defects. The disease clusters are occurring in communities near toxic pollution. Childhood asthma is covered below; childhood cancer and birth defect disease clusters are in succeeding chapters.

Childhood Asthma

In May 2005 the EPA and CDC released the following information regarding childhood asthma:

- "Asthma is the most common serious chronic disease of childhood.
- Asthma is the third-ranking cause of hospitalization among children under 15.
- Asthma in children is the cause of almost five million physician visits and more than 200,000 hospitalizations.
- Asthma accounts for one-third of all pediatric emergency room visits and is the fourth-most common cause of pediatric visits to the doctor's office.
- An average of one out of every 13 school-age children has asthma.
- Asthma is the leading cause of school absenteeism from a chronic childhood condition. 14.7 million school days are missed each year due to asthma."

Asthma is caused by chronic inflammation of the respiratory airways with episodes of reversible airway obstruction. This causes swelling of the lining of the airway, tightening of respiratory muscles and increased secretion of mucus. Symptoms of an asthma attack include coughing, wheezing, shortness of breath and chest tightness. The attacks are terrifying to the children and their parents, as a child struggles to breath. It is a chronic disease with exacerbations and can be life threatening if not managed properly.

Studies have shown that asthma can be triggered by exposure to allergens like animal dander, dust mites, mold, and cockroach droppings. Synthetic floor rugs and pressed wood furniture can release toxic vapors in the home. Secondhand tobacco smoke is also believed to trigger attacks. As mentioned earlier, insecticides and chemicals used in the home are most frequently reported to be responsible for the growing number of both children and adults with asthma.

Millions of children live in areas where industries violate pollution laws and pollute the environment with sulfur dioxide and fine particulate soot. Power plants and industries expel this matter into the air and water close to where children live and attend school. Studies have shown that the greater the pollution in an area, the higher the incidence of childhood asthma. Not only is there an increase in the number of new asthma cases, but there is also an increase in attacks among children who already have asthma.

Public health advocacy groups feel that a fully operational national disease tracking network could find the number of cases of asthma and their location. Then, hopefully, common disease triggers could be found in the areas of high asthma incidence. This could lead to better treatments and possibly a cure. A few states do track asthma incidence, some states do a poor job at tracking, but most states don't track asthma at all.

Chapter 14

Childhood Disease Clusters-Cancer

It is devastating when children are diagnosed with cancer. The entire family suffers when a child must undergo chemotherapy and radiation treatments. Siblings can feel ignored. Mothers and fathers can become overwhelmed trying to juggle work, family, and hospital visits, and this too often leads to divorce. Children with cancer miss a lot of school, when they return other students may treat them differently, and this can affect their self esteem. The good news is that more children are surviving cancer as a result of advances in treatments. The bad news is that children continue to be diagnosed with cancer. We can look at a few such clusters, but let's first look at some cancer statistics.

The following is a 2003 report provided TFAH (Trust For Americas Health). This information found at the TFAH website was compiled from data obtained from the National Cancer Institute and the American Cancer Society.

"Survival rates for childhood cancer have risen sharply over the past 20 years. In the United States, more than 75 percent of children with cancer are alive five years after diagnosis, compared with about 60 percent in the mid-1970s. Much of this dramatic improvement is due to the development of improved therapies for children's cancer. However, there are a number of childhood cancer-related statistics that are troubling. These statistics include:

- Brain Cancer and other tumors in children's nervous systems rose more than 25% between 1973 and 1996.
- Over the past 20 years, there have been some increases in the incidence of children diagnosed with all forms of invasive cancer; from 11.4 cases per 100,000 children in 1975 to 15.2 per 100,000 children in 1998.
- Leukemia, which is the most common childhood cancer, increased by more than 15% over the past 20 years. Most of the increase in leukemia rates in the past 20 years has been in a kind of cancer called acute lymphoblastic leukemia or ALL."

The TFAH report continues with the following information:

"A recent study in the American Journal of Public health reported an association between household chemicals and ALL. According to the Children's Cancer Group Epidemiology Program, a network of pediatric epidemiologists, children are 5 to 6 times more likely to develop leukemia and brain cancer if their families use pesticides at home. There are realistic concerns about childrens' exposure to solvents in the home. These solvents are used for refinishing furniture, or building models."

Chronic Disease / Pollution Connection

Toms River, New Jersey Childhood Cancer

Toms River, New Jersey is one of those disease clusters where cancer rates in children were increasing in the 1990's. The New Jersey Department of Health performed a health study in 1996. The study found that between 1979 and 1995, ninety children were diagnosed with cancer. The incidence of leukemia, brain, and central nervous system cancers were much higher than expected.

Parents sought help for their children at nearby cancer centers. Mothers who met at Memorial Sloan Kettering Cancer Center in New York City were shocked to find out they all lived in the same Toms River area and all had children being treated for cancer. They started a support group for dealing with the devastation of having a child with cancer.

In 1995, a nurse at Children's Hospital in Philadelphia, Pennsylvania became concerned about the number of childhood cancer patients she was seeing from the Toms River area. She called the EPA and the state health department was notified. A government study of the affected children found contaminated well water and toxic air emission from nearby chemical factories. The wells were found to be contaminated by waste seeping into the water supply from more than 45,000 drums of chemicals belonging to a nearby chemical factory.

The New Jersey Department of Health and ATSDR performed a health study in the Toms River area. Their reported conclusions in 1997 provided the following information:

"The study failed to find any single risk factor responsible for the rise in childhood cancer. An association was found between prenatal exposure to contaminated water and leukemia in female children. Also an association was found between prenatal exposure to the air from the chemical plants and leukemia in female children diagnosed prior to age five."

In December 2001 the media reported that the chemical companies and the local water company agreed to a multi-million dollar settlement for 69 families. They did this without admitting blame. The money was said to be of little consolation to the families, especially to 15 families whose children had died.

Fallon, Nevada Leukemia Cluster

Fallon, Nevada is the location of a childhood leukemia cluster. Fallon is a military and farming community with a population of 8,300 about sixty miles from Reno. My story about Fallon focuses on one mother named Brenda, who I have met, and her son Dustin. Dustin was diagnosed in 1999 with Acute Lymphocytic Leukemia (ALL) at age three. Brenda had noticed Dustin was listless and when she discovered bruises over parts of his body she rushed him to the Emergency Room. Blood tests pointed to leukemia. Twice, Dustin was flown to Sacramento, California for chemotherapy, requiring a month's stay each time. Dustin's blood work has to be watched closely and he continues to take many medications, but he was considered to be in remission. His parents looked forward to that fifth year that doctors consider a cure date.

Dustin was the second case of leukemia in the small community. The first child had been diagnosed with leukemia after his father took him to see a physician when he noticed that his child was weak and listless. The doctor found a large tumor in the child's chest. He underwent two courses of chemotherapy, two bone marrow transplants, and radiation therapy. The treatments were unsuccessful and several weeks later he died.

Within two years the number of leukemia cases in Fallon climbed to sixteen. All the children had the same type of acute lymphoblastic leukemia (ALL), except one child who had acute myelogenous leukemia (AML).

The families wondered what could be in their environment that could cause the leukemia. One possibility considered was arsenic in the water that occurs naturally as a result of the area's geology. Could it be pesticides sprayed on farm crops? Could it be connected to the Fallon Naval Air Station and the jet fuel that runs in a pipeline under their community? Could it be lingering fallout from 1960 underground nuclear testing?

Brenda became an advocate for the children in Fallon. She formed an organization called "Families In Search of Truth" (FIST). She wrote and/or called the Nevada State Health Department, the CDC, the EPA, and her state and federal legislators. She spoke about Fallon's problem at community meetings, at state legislative meetings, and at U.S. Senate hearings. It took a year for the Nevada State Health Department to respond to requests for help. By then two children had died.

The Nevada State Health Department and the CDC conducted studies on the children involved. The Nevada State Health Department had to first "develop a protocol for the collection of specimens, secure clinical space for testing, train a team to collect samples and procure commitments from environmental laboratories to examine field samples".

This provides an example of how state health departments are unprepared to efficiently track diseases for a much-needed national disease tracking network or to manage a bioterrorism attack in this country.

In the summer of 2002 the CDC found that 80% of the people tested in Fallon had high levels of tungsten and arsenic in their urine. The Nevada State Health Department requested that the ATSDR join them in examining health concerns in Fallon. The ATSDR released the following information in a press release February 12, 2003:

- "The ATSDR did not find a relationship between environmental exposure pathways and the leukemia cases in Churchill County.
- Evidence cross checked by multiple regulatory agencies showed no evidence of leaks from the JP-8 fuel pipeline serving Naval Air Station Fallon.
- Activities at the Naval Air Station are not a public health hazard.
- Eating the mercury-contaminated fish and duck found in Churchill County is a potential public health hazard for humans, especially for long-term exposures to young children and women of childbearing age. County residents should follow the Nevada State Health Department health advisories for fish and ducks.
- The results of tap water samples collected in 2002 from seventy six homes showed high levels of naturally occurring metals, such as arsenic and uranium. Tap water from these homes is drawn from private and municipal wells. The sampling results reflect water quality from the three different groundwater sources used for drinking water.

- Arsenic levels in many tap water samples substantially exceeded the recently revised U.S.EPA drinking water standard for arsenic. Because studies in other parts of the world indicate that long-term exposures to similar levels of arsenic in drinking water can be associated with a number of adverse health effects, ATSDR recommends that currently, tap water in Churchill County not be used as a primary drinking water source.

- Uranium levels in tap water from some shallow private wells substantially exceeded the EPA drinking water standard for uranium. Toxicologic studies indicate that long-term exposures to uranium in drinking water at these concentrations may pose an increased risk of kidney damage. Therefore, people using those wells should consider using alternate sources for drinking water to reduce their exposures.

- Tungsten was found in most tap water samples collected. The EPA has no drinking water standard for tungsten. Research on the possible toxicologic effects of tungsten is very limited. However, efforts are underway to further define tungsten exposures in Nevada and to evaluate potential routes of exposure."

Why are levels of some toxic substances so high in the Fallon area, and how long have these high levels existed? One researcher found that trees can shed light on how long they have existed. Apparently trees record information about environmental conditions that can be found in their annual growth rings. Researchers compared metal concentration patterns in the rings for the past five years with those from a five-year period when leukemia rates were normal. They found that tungsten levels had risen and that there was no detectable change in the level of any other metal.

Public health studies have not found a reason why so many children in Fallon have leukemia. Fallon residents want additional research to examine potential links between chemical exposures and chronic diseases. Brenda did not accept what she has been told. She again went to Capital Hill to speak to legislators about the problems in her community and the need for a fully operational chronic disease tracking network. She has continued to seek support from the scientific community to find answers for the leukemia in Fallon. Brenda is a wonderful role model for all of us.

Chapter 15

Childhood Disease Clusters - Birth Defects

Another serious childhood disease cluster problem found in the US today is birth defects. The Center for Disease Control and Prevention reports the following regarding birth defects:

"Birth defects are the leading cause of infant mortality in the United States, accounting for more than 20% of all infant deaths. About 120,000 U.S. babies are born each year with birth defects and 8,000 die during their first year of life. In addition, birth defects are the fifth-leading cause of years of potential life lost and contributes substantially to childhood morbidity and long-term disability."

The CDC provides a great deal more information on birth defects at their website. Some highlights from the site include the following information:

- "The most common birth defect identified is heart defects. About 1 in every 100 to 200 babies is born with a heart defect. Heart defects make up about

103

one-third to one-fourth of all birth defects. Some of these heart defects can be serious, and a few are very severe. In some places of the world, heart defects cause half of all deaths from birth defects in children less than I year of age.

- Neural tube defects which are defects of the spine (spina bifida) and brain (anencephaly). They affect 1of 1,000 pregnancies. These defects can be serious and are often life threatening. They happen less often than heart defects, but they cause many fetal and infant deaths.

- Birth defects of the lip and roof of the mouth are also common. These defects, known as orofacial clefts, include cleft lip, cleft palate, and combined cleft lip and palate. Cleft lip is more common than cleft palate. In many places in the world, orofacial clefts defects affect about 1 in 700 to 1,000 babies.

- Other defects are common but rarely life threatening though they often require medical and surgical attention. An example is hypospadias, a fairly common defect found in male babies. In babies with hypospadias, the opening of the urethra (where urine comes out) is not on the tip of the penis but on the underside."

The two neural tube defects reported by the CDC were spina bifida, which is failure of the spinal canal to close properly, and anencephaly which is the absence of all or part of the brain. You will hear about these defects being reported in disease clusters across the country. Both genetics and environmental factors are suspected to cause birth defects. Environmental exposures to toxic chemicals and radiation are commonly found in birth defect clusters. Unfortunately, the impacts of most toxic chemicals on a developing child have not been evaluated. The cause of 60 to 70% of birth defects is unknown. Researchers are alarmed by so many birth defect clusters and are said to be committed to finding answers.

Florida Birth Defects Cluster

Escambia and Santa Rosa counties had Superfund hazardous waste sites believed to have exposed people to heavy concentrations of toxic chemicals for many years. Escambia County ranks 22nd out of 3300 counties nationwide in the amount of toxic releases reported by the EPA at that time.

Escambia and Santa Rosa counties had elevated rates of birth defects in 2001. It has been reported that Escambia ranks 38th among U.S. counties in the release of neurotoxicants and developmental toxins that have been shown to damage the way a child's body and brain develops, and have been linked to numerous birth defects and learning disabilities.

Death rates from all forms of cancer in Escambia and Santa Rosa counties also far exceeded national rates. Public health and environmental officials found elevated rates of brain, liver, kidney and lung cancer rates among people living in the area.

Federal regulators reportedly suspect dioxin, arsenic, lead and mercury contamination from the area's superfund sites and manufacturing plants as causes for the problems in Santa Rosa and Escambia counties. The University of West Florida announced in June 2004 that the Center for Environmental Diagnostics and Bioremediation Department would be conducting several studies in Northwest Florida to identify threats to public health. The studies were commissioned by appropriations from Congress. Collaborative studies were to be performed with the Georgia Institute of Technology conducting air quality studies in the region. Other environmental studies to be performed include evaluations of people living near a Superfund site in Escambia County and of children exhibiting elevated lead levels. Look for results in the media.

Autism Disease Clusters

Some conditions not previously recognized as birth defects are increasingly being viewed by scientists as birth defects today. Autism is one of those birth defects. Autism is a severe developmental disorder in which children appear to be isolated from the world around them. Common problems are poor language skills and an inability to handle social relations. Parents describe their autistic child as a child who seems to be in their own little world and not connecting with anyone in their environment. They are often perceived as being withdrawn. Treatment involves behavioral therapy and some children are helped by medication. There is no known cause or cure.

An autism disease cluster is located in Brick Township, New Jersey. Brick Township is thirty miles east of Trenton, New Jersey. There were a reported seventy five children with autism in Brick Township. Four families in fact, were said to have more than one child with autism.

The EPA confirmed that the groundwater beneath the Brick Township landfill is contaminated with hazardous substances. In an EPA report on the Brick Township Landfill dated February 2004 the following information was reported:

"Approximately 3,000 people lived within a 1 mile radius of the site. Ground water is the source of public and private drinking supplies for 58,000 people living within a 3 mile radius of the site. Samplings taken at the site showed that 67 substances exceeded Ground Water Quality Standards. The removal of drums and filling and venting of seepage pits has greatly reduced the potential for exposure to contaminated materials."

The Brick Township cleanup continues. Large toxic waste site cleanup history has shown that this process can take decades to complete.

About the same time that New Jersey was experiencing what was considered a high incidence of autism, the State of California was also experiencing elevated numbers. A report on autism and possible environmental exposures was published by New York Mount Sinai School of Medicine, Center for Children's Health and the Environment. The report found an increase in autism world-wide but questioned the increased numbers reported for the United States. The report did point out concerns about autism in the state of California, finding an increase in the number of parents using the special services available for autistic children. There was a 210% increase in the number of people seeking assistance between 1987 and 1998.

Autism research is now being conducted at the University of California Davis. Possible causes being studied are maternal age, genetics, vaccinations, and environmental factors.

Chapter 16

The Military Base/Disease Cluster Connection

Military bases seem to appear too often in chronic disease clusters. Both the South Weymouth area of Massachusetts and Fallon, Nevada have disease clusters surrounding military bases. JP8 jet fuel has been suggested as a possible source of the disease cluster illnesses in both communities. Looking into JP8 jet fuel has revealed some surprising information and led to my finding a more widespread problem.

The Pentagon uses JP8 fuel as a universal battlefield fuel, capable of powering trucks, tanks, airplanes, and even infantry stoves. But military personnel and people living near air bases can reportedly be exposed to a super fine mist or aerosol of unburned JP8 fuel that is produced by the plane engines as they warm-up and during takeoff. Jets are reported to also dump fuel in flight.

JP8 fuel consists of a complex mixture of hydrocarbons, including polyaromatic hydrocarbons and benzene, a known carcinogen. There was an ALS disease cluster of 127 cases found in 2000 at Kelly Air Force Base in San Antonio, Texas. This high occurrence of ALS was among former and current workers at the Air Force Base. The high numbers of ALS cases baffled experts. At that time there was an ongoing environmental cleanup and the Air Force was conducting Health Risks Studies.

The Air Force risk studies later found no connection between the base and the ALS disease cluster. The ATSDR also performed a health consultation at Kelly Air Force Base. Their study was published March 5, 2002. The study did not find a link between metal exposure or organic chemical exposure and ALS. This was said to be due to lack of well characterized evaluation of past exposure.

A research paper in 2000 titled, "Immunotoxicology of JP-8 Jet Fuel", was written by Dr. David T. Harris at Arizona University, Tucson. It provides very important information regarding JP8 jet fuel and health. Dr.Harris's research provides the following information:

> "Chronic jet fuel exposure could be detrimental to Air Force personnel, not only by adversely affecting their work performance but also by predisposing these individuals to increased incidences of infectious disease and cancer. Chronic exposure to jet fuel has been shown to adversely affect human liver function, to cause emotional dysfunction, to cause abnormal electroencephalograms, to cause shortened attention spans, and to decrease sensorimotor speed. Currently, there are no standards for personnel exposure to jet fuels of any kind, let alone JP-8 jet fuel. Kerosene based petroleum distillates have been associated with hepatic, renal, neurologic and pulmonary toxicity in animals models and human

occupational exposures. The U.S. Department of Labor, Bureau of Labor Statistics estimates that over 1.3 million workers were exposed to jet fuels in 1992. Thus, jet fuel exposure may not only have serious consequences for USAF personnel, but also may have potential harmful effects upon a significant number of civilian workers. Short-term (7 day) JP-8 jet fuel exposure causes lung injury - - - ."

Dr. Harris continues and reports the following regarding long term effects of JP8 jet fuel exposure:

"Long-term exposures, although demonstrating evidence of lung recovery, results in injury to secondary organs such as liver, kidneys and spleen."

There is a reported leukemia and immune deficiency disease cluster at a Coast Guard Base in San Diego, California. It is at the end of a runway used by both military aircraft, and civilian aircraft powered by Jet-A fuel, which is similar to JP-8. Another childhood leukemia cluster has been confirmed in Sierra Vista, Arizona, which is home to the military airfield at Fort Huachuca. This is similar to the leukemia cluster reported earlier in Fallon, Nevada, which is also near air bases. Scientists have begun looking at jet fuel as a possible common finding.

In August 1998 the ATSDR released a public health statement for Jet Fuel JP-5 and JP-8 which began with the following information:

"This public health statement tells you about the jet fuels JP-5 and JP-8 and the effects of exposure. The Environmental Protection Agency (EPA) identifies the most hazardous waste sites in the nation.

These sites make up the National Priorities List (NPL) and are the sites targeted for long-term federal cleanup activities. JP-5 and JP-8 have been found in at least 22 of the 1,445 current or former NPL sites. However, the total number of NPL sites evaluated for this substance is not known. As more sites are evaluated, the sites at which JP-5 and JP-8 are found may increase. This information is important because exposure to these substances may harm you and because these sites may be sources of exposure - - -."

You may read the entire very informative report at the ATSDR website identified in this book's bibliography

Disease clusters and jet fuel exposure are also being addressed in other countries. A report from Italy identified a leukemia cluster among troops who used JP-8 while fighting in Bosnia. Several research studies are being performed in the United Kingdom on possible harmful effects of jet fuel on human health in that country. The U.S. government continues to investigate the possible adverse effects of jet fuel or any other contamination at military bases. Government officials report that there is no proven connection between JP8 jet fuel and disease clusters.

Chapter 17

Many Other Disease Clusters

Many more disease clusters are located throughout the United States. The list that follows gives you a brief look at some of the many other disease clusters identified in this country. I am certain that there are many more disease clusters not yet recognized by public health officials.

- **Anniston, Alabama**
  Community and surrounding area suffered from very elevated rates of rare cancers, birth defects, neurological diseases, asthma, kidney disease, and liver disease. The county is home to a former munitions depot which closed in 1995, an ironworks, a toxic waste incinerator, and an industrial coolant manufacturer. The community successfully sued a local industry for health damage to residents.

- **Bronx, New York**
  There was a high incidence of cancer and birth defects near a toxic landfill. No environmental connections had been reported at that time.

- **Brownsville, Texas**

    There were 9,636 cases with one or more birth defects over the last 20 years. The polluted Rio Grande River was the suspected contamination source.

- **Cape Cod, Massachusetts**

    Breast cancer rates were 20% higher than rest of Massachusetts from 1982-1994. Water supply contamination suspected.

- **Cedar Rapids, Iowa**

    Ninety cancer and forty four precancerous conditions were diagnosed in graduates of Regis High School, (eight cases of cancer and five precancerous conditions in one class of 113 students). Nearby superfund site and heavy nuclear fallout were suspected causes.

- **Charleston County, South Carolina**

    Higher than expected cases of colon, stomach, rectal, lung, larynx, and pleural cancer. Asbestos exposure is the suspected cause.

- **Chesterfield County, Virginia**

    Elevated oral cancer and respiratory cancer reported at the Department of Defense General Supply Center, a military supply distributor with a toxic dump site in the area.

- **Columbiana County, Ohio**

    There were reports of elevated rates of cancer, Parkinson's, and Crohn's disease rates in this area near a chemical plant Superfund site. The chemicals Mirex and Photomirex were found in the blood of fourteen of forty two workers.

- **DePue, Illinois**

    Elevated numbers of MS cases near a zinc smelting plant. Studies found elevated levels of heavy metals in soil, water, and air. No environmental connection was made.

- **Dickson County, Tennessee**

    Between 1997 and 2000, eighteen children were born with a cleft lip or cleft palate. TCE and Toluene chemical releases suspected source of problem.

- **East Hampton, New York**

    Contains a disease cluster of young people who graduated from East Hampton High from 1990 to 1997. Ten people have been diagnosed with lymphoma and other cancers. All were diagnosed within a period of a little over one year. Exposure to radiation leaks from a nuclear power plants suspected but not proven.

- **Elmira, NY**

    Since the late 1970s, at least 40 students have been diagnosed with cancer. Thirteen cases were diagnosed in a recent three-year period. The school was built on top of the previous location of a heavily polluted industrial company. Investigations were ongoing.

- **Fairfield, Maine**

    A high incidence of brain cancer reported near a toxic landfill site.

- **Fernald, Ohio**

    Elevated death rates due to Hodgkin's disease in 4,014 uranium processing workers between 1951 and 1989. This town is near a nuclear plant.

- **Geauga County, Ohio**

    In an area with 152 homes, residents documented 142 people with cancer that have lived there in the last twenty years. A motor transit company is said to have buried two toxic-fluid-filled tankers on land adjoining the housing area.

- **Gelena, Kansas**

    Community has reports of chronic kidney disease, stroke, heart disease, and skin cancer in a population exposed to toxic metals (lead and cadmium) near a mining toxic dump site.

- **Greenport, Brooklyn, New York**

    Elevated rates of cancer, lupus, and asthma found in the vicinity of a large sewage treatment plant.

- **Hanford, Washington**

    Elevated incidence of various cancers and thyroid diseases near Hanford Nuclear Reservation. This facility was reported to have released radiation and chemicals into the environment for past fifty years. No environmental connection made.

- **Hardemann County, Tennessee**

    Contains a liver disease cluster among residents exposed to solvents from a toxic waste dump.

- **Hazelton and Corry, Pennsylvania**

    High incidences of prostate cancer, stomach cancer, and leukemia in Hazel Township. Environmental officials found 50,000 gallons of gasoline leaking into soil and into abandoned mines under the homes.

- **Herculaneum, Jefferson County, Missouri**

    Elevated numbers of MS and ALS cases. Also elevated levels of lead in blood samples of adults and in 28% of the children. Location of a lead smelting plant. Ongoing study was to be completed 2005.

- **Laredo, Texas**

    High incidence of several types of cancer reported. Brownfields and ozone pollution from industries were suspected causes.

- **Los Alamos County, New Mexico**

    Excessive thyroid cancer cases and brain cancer cases in surrounding communities. Suspected radiation exposure from Los Alamos National Laboratory. Town's water supply wells tested positive for tritium and strontium-90.

- **Louisville, Kentucky**

    Very elevated rates of lung, brain, liver, and childhood cancer were reported in the area near a complex of chemical companies.

- **Maryvale, Arizona**

    Residents identified forty nine leukemia cases over twenty one years. Jet fuel exposure from the nearby military base was suspected. The Arizona Department of health took ten years to investigate and found no environmental connection.

- **Middletown, Iowa**

    Workers at Iowa Army Ammunition Plant have pulmonary cancer rates several times higher than rest of the state from 1969 to 1999. Liver cancer was fourteen times higher in these workers than the rest of the state. Also elevated cancer rates in residents of Middletown and West Burlington.

- **North Haven, New Haven County, Connecticut**

    Several dozen cases of a rare brain cancer were reported among workers at a jet-engine manufacturing company. An ongoing study was reported to tentatively be completed in 2008.

- **Oak Ridge, Tennessee**

    Nearly 100 Oakwood residents have been diagnosed with thyroid cancer and brain damage. Suspected toxic releases from nuclear weapons plant, uranium plant and research facility.

- **Pampa, Texas**

    Higher than expected numbers of Down's syndrome and leukemia cases were reported. The cause was suspected to be toxic emissions from a pharmaceutical plant.

- **Portsmouth, Ohio**

    An elevated death rate due to Hodgkin's disease among 8,887 workers at nuclear facility between 1954 and 1991. No environmental connection proven.

- **Rochester, New York**

    Eleven workers at a manufacturing plant developed MS between 1970 and 1979. Zinc exposure was suspected.

- **San Francisco, California**

    ALS was diagnosed in three members of the 49ers football team in the 1980s. (There may be a football connection; in Britain, the Football Association launched a study after a number of soccer players died from ALS in 2001; In Italy, 40 soccer players died from ALS from 1960 to 1996). No environmental connection made.

- **San Jose, California**

    There have been hundreds of cases of lymph, blood, brain, and breast cancer, and also multiple myeloma reported in the Silicon Valley. Exposure to trichloroethylene, cadmium, toluene, benzene, and arsenic in the workplace was suspected cause.

- **San Miguel County, New Mexico**

    Very elevated cancer rates located near three Superfund sites, many Brownfields, and thirty six polluting industries. ATSDR consultation concluded that there was an indeterminate public health hazard.

- **Shoalwater Bay Indian Reservation, Washington State**

    Higher than expected miscarriage and still birth rate, but no conclusive environmental connection was made.

- **Sierra Vista, Arizona**

    This is a town with six childhood leukemia cases living within half a mile of the U.S. Fort Huachuca Army Base airfield runway. A potential jet fuel connection remained unproven. An ATSDR study could find no environmental connection.

- **Silver Valley, Idaho**

    This area had high cancer rates. A Superfund site with mining operations was believed to have polluted the area with arsenic, lead, and other toxicants.

- **Simi Valley, California**

    Propulsion Laboratory employees and family members had higher than normal cancer rates. State Health Department detected elevated bladder cancer rates within a 5 mile radius of the Propulsion facility. No conclusive environmental connection was reported.

- **South Boston, Massachusetts**

    This area had twenty six cases of scleroderma and sixty cases of lupus. There is a possible link to industrial solvent exposure. The Massachusetts State Health Department was conducting a study.

- **South Texas border**

    Seventy four women who lived in the Texas border counties gave birth to children with severe birth defects from 1993 through early 1995. Thirty six babies were born with spina bifida (opening in the spine), thirty four with anencephaly (minimal or no brain development), and four with encephalocele (protrusion of the brain through the skull). Pesticide residues and industrial chemicals in the soil are suspected causes.

- **South Weber, Utah**

  Their brain cancer disease cluster was said to be statistically significant. There was a questionable link to an incinerator found to exceed federal emissions standards for dioxin.

- **St. Lucie and St. Martin Counties, Florida**

  Thirty children in St. Lucie County and twelve in St. Martin County were diagnosed with rare brain cancer and nerve-cell cancers. The suspected chemical exposures link had not been proven.

- **State of Colorado**

  5500 people have MS throughout the state. One in 800 Coloradans has MS. Studies were unable to identify a cause.

- **Suffolk County, New York**

  Elevated lung cancer rates prompted a study by the NY State Health Department. An asbestos exposure link was questioned.

- **Sugar Creek, Missouri**

  In addition to an MS cluster, the community also has a brain cancer cluster located near a petroleum refinery. Studies found no environmental connection.

- **Tucson, Arizona**

  There were elevated birth defects among children born to families living in part of the city where the water supply was reportedly contaminated with industrial solvents.

- **Waldridge, Ohio**

  A leukemia disease cluster of ten individuals was reported. Five cases who resided within a five mile radius of each other were diagnosed within a three month period. Questionable cause was lead exposure from industry.

- **Washington County, Ohio (Marietta area)**
  Elevated cancer rates have been reported. Industrial air pollution was found to be ten times higher than expected.

- **Washington State**
  6500 people with MS live in central and western parts of the state. Studies were being performed.

The disease clusters that have been mentioned all have similar stories of families fighting for their health and/or that of their children. The affected people, their families, and neighbors must educate themselves about chemicals they can't even pronounce. They have to become knowledgeable about disease processes and treatments, as well as state and federal laws, in order to deal with agencies paid to protect them, but often unwilling or unable to do so.

Chapter 18

Why Disease Cluster Studies Fail

Disease cluster investigations are being conducted all over the United States. The results are typically very disappointing. The communities that I have mentioned fight to obtain help from their health departments. Years go by and often only persistent disease cluster activists get any recognition from their public health agencies. Health studies consistently find no environmental connections, even though nearby industries are found to be emitting toxic chemicals into disease cluster neighborhoods.

Over 1000 calls are reportedly made to public health officials each year from people concerned about a high incidence of a disease in their neighborhoods. People receive varying kinds of responses. The public health system management of disease cluster reports is in need of considerable improvement. The following research data provides insight into the problem.

An excellent research report by Tony Dutzik and Jeremiah Baumann was published September 2002, titled, "Health Tracking and Disease Clusters, The Lack of Data on

Chronic Disease Incidence and Its Impact on Disease Cluster Investigations". It was published jointly by the U.S. Public Interest Research Group (PIRG) Education Fund, and the PennEnvironment Research and Policy Center. The report provides answers to questions about disease cluster investigations that have been very troubling for years. Public health agencies were surveyed by the research group, and the responses that had been given by the public health agencies to the disease cluster members were recorded. Those responses varied depending on the state agency involved. The responses found in the research report are listed below:

- "A few agencies reported no process for responding to disease cluster reports.
- Several said they emphasized life style causes for diseases, like smoking, as the reason for disease cluster.
- Some agencies required people to fill out ten to twenty pages of information, the forms that were returned were used to collect epidemiological information, but the agencies had little or no staff to pursue further action.
- A few agencies said they would not follow up unless people either showed sufficient interest to return forms or had their elected representatives contact them to request investigations.
- The scope of studies is often unduly expanded. Investigators must determine, in the early point in their analysis, the spatial and temporal boundaries of the community they intend to study. Where a hypothesis as to the cause of a disease cluster exists, health officials should use the hypothesis as the basis of their boundary setting decisions. Yet, such decisions are inherently judgment calls and

open the possibility for intentional or unwitting distortion. A cluster of disease that is limited to the area around a source of air pollution, for example, can be made to statistically disappear if public health authorities choose to use broad swaths of territory, such as a county as the basis for their analysis."

This is the answer to the questionable practice used by public health agencies when they expand the study areas. They usually include entire townships or county populations, rather than just the smaller community where the disease cluster is located. This is a common practice in Ohio as well as a few other states.

The research report continues telling us the following;

- "Multiple diseases in an area are often not included in studies. In addition, public health officials often determine which illnesses suspected by a community are studied and which aren't. Because many requests for disease cluster investigations include several diseases suspected to be in excess, limiting the number of diseases under study could lead to some potential disease clusters being ignored."

An example of multiple diseases reported but not included in a study may have occurred in Middlefield, Ohio.

The Study in Middlefield, Ohio

Middlefield is a village of less than 2000 people, which includes a large Amish population. People in the village were being diagnosed with neurological problems, liver and kidney cancer, and birth defects at an alarming rate. Middlefield is also the home of a rubber factory. The rubber product company became a concern to the residents because of their history of non-compliance with EPA standards. The people felt it could be the cause of the illnesses. According to residents, letters and calls were made to the OEPA as far back as 1967 but to no avail.

I was able to contact Ron, a Middlefield resident who is working to find a reason for the health problems in Middlefield. Ron grew up near the rubber factory site. He worked as post master for many years in the community before he was forced to retire at age 38 because of failing health. Ron told me that he was diagnosed with peripheral neuropathy, a neurological condition that causes numbness, weakness, and pain in various parts of the body, especially the extremities. When he sought professional help, he said his physician suspected heavy metal poisoning. Lab work verified that his blood did contain chromium, cadmium, and strontium at levels high enough to cause damage to nerve endings.

Residents continued to look for help from OEPA with no success. Out of frustration, Ron's wife Laura wrote a letter to then Vice President Al Gore in February 1994. Within two months, a team from the U.S.EPA arrived to investigate. They took water and soil samples from the factory sites which showed elevated levels of the metals chromium and strontium. Then an employee informed inspectors about a concrete walled basin in a factory that was full of sludge. The basin contained high levels of the toxic chemicals tetrachlorothene, chromium and lead. Test showed that the toxic sludge had spread off-site. Eventually, the company paid to have the basin cleaned and sealed. Even though the U.S.EPA knew about the chemicals migrating off-site, they concluded that there was no imminent danger and gave the site to the OEPA for cleanup. This was expected to take 2 to 20 years.

Middlefield residents were also concerned about the health problems in the village. So they contacted the ODH for help in finding out what was causing the neurological problems, the kidney and liver cancers, and the birth defects in their community. A representative from the ODH later announced that he would look at the cancer problems in Middlefield. He said the residents only asked for cancer studies. <u>But the residents strongly disagreed, saying they asked for a study of all the disease conditions in Middlefield.</u>

The ODH study results were presented to Middlefield citizens in February 2004. The cancer study had been unfortunately expanded to include all of Middlefield Township. It looked at cancer cases in the township and the village from 1996 to 2000. The results found fewer cases of leukemia than expected in males and more cases of leukemia than expected in females, based on national cancer incidence. No environmental connection was found between the cancer cases and the local rubber factory toxic waste.

The ODH reported high levels of manganese, a naturally occurring substance, in township wells. They recommended that home owners install water softeners to take care of the problem. Studies have found that long-term exposure to high levels of manganese could cause central nervous system damage.

In the spring of 2005 the OEPA was slowly still cleaning up the contamination around the factory site by pulling contaminants from the soil, processing them and releasing them into the air. Ron and a clergy group were fighting to get all the sites cleaned up more rapidly because of the continuing health problems. Residents reportedly can tell you about a house where all the children had leukemia; a house where three sisters had cancer of the uterus; and a family where the children had heart defects. And then Ron's wife, Laura, was diagnosed with a peripheral neuropathy. Ron's mother-in-law, who lived about a block from the rubber factory site, was diagnosed with ALS and died. An aunt who worked at the rubber factory died from brain cancer, and Ron's brother was having neurological problems.

Then, Laura found carbon black in the rubber factory parking lot that had spread into the adjacent neighborhood. This supported their suspicion that the factory continued to spread contamination into the neighboring community. The carbon was found to contain polychlorinated biphenyls (PCBs) in amounts warranting the U.S.EPA to do further studies at the factory site. PCBs can cause cancers, developmental problems, and damage to immune systems. Still, in 2005 the residents continued to seek answers and hoped to soon have a clean environment to live in.

The Health Tracking & Disease Cluster Research study also pointed to another significant problem about chronic diseases cluster studies.

> "The cluster investigations are hampered by lack of data on the rate of a disease that would be expected in any given community."

That certainly was the case in Wellington, Ohio, when the state health department reported that a Prevalence Study had to be done first to find the expected rate for the disease before the MS incidence could be addressed. What happened in Galion, Ohio is another example.

Galion, Ohio

Galion, population 12,391, is about sixty miles southwest of Wellington. A suspected elevated incidence of MS was reported there in the early 1980s. In 1982, the Ohio Department of Health, responding to concerned citizens requests, began collecting names of the local MS patients. Nothing happened for five years and Galion residents were reportedly informed that the paperwork had been lost. Consequently, the study did not begin until 1987. At that time, the suspected sources of the MS cases in Galion were the nearby Olentangy River, and industrial sites including an ironworks plant established in 1907.

In 1984, the OEPA came to Galion and told local industries to stop discharging metal waste into the river. Families were also told to stop using the sludge from a local sewage treatment plant for fertilizers on their farm fields. A sample of river water detected cadmium, copper, and chromium, all at elevated levels. Chromium and cadmium are known to be very toxic. The OEPA was concerned about a fish kill in a pond fed by Olentangy River, but at the time didn't see it as any risk or danger to people.

Residents reported that a twenty nine year old man was diagnosed with MS a year after two of his high school classmates were diagnosed. They lived on the same block of Fairview Avenue in Galion. They reportedly were born within eighteen months of each other, diagnosed within eighteen months of each other, and were very supportive of each other.

In 1991, the ODH published the results of the study of the Galion MS disease cluster. Just as in Wellington, they had expanded the study to include all of Polk Township residents.

Under this study, the ODH eliminated eight suspected cases because they did not have the disease or lived outside the study area. Another eight cases could not be located or died. A resident involved in initiating the study felt that 50+ people had a Galion MS connection. But some time had passed before the ODH performed their study and some residents had died or moved away. <u>Did expanding the geographical area of the study make a difference?</u>

The ODH concluded that, with a population of less than 15,000 people, the Galion area could expect twenty cases under the National MS Society statistics. Considering the expanded area, Galion didn't qualify as a disease cluster. The ODH also reported that blood studies performed on MS patients did not show excessive levels of heavy metals. The people in Galion with MS were angered and dismayed, but they felt that they had done all they could do.

The ODH probably worked with some very real disadvantages when they performed the health study in Galion. They had to work with what tools were available for disease cluster studies at that time. Did they have methods and procedures for performing an MS health study in the late 80's? Did they have information about the expected prevalence of MS? Keep in mind that this data was still being developed for the Wellington MS cluster in 2002-2005. You will see the same prevalence information being developed today in other disease cluster studies across the United States.

I found another Galion research report titled "Disease Clustering of Multiple Sclerosis In Galion, Ohio 1982-1985" by T. Ingalls, School of Public Health, Boston University School of Medicine, Massachusetts. The Ingalls research article was at the National Library of Medicine, National Institute of Health, and National Center for Biotechnology Information computer site. He reported the following:

> "Epidemiological evidence indicates that the outbreak of 30 to 40 cases of multiple sclerosis and other demyelization syndromes (damage to the body's nerve fibers) in Galion, Ohio, USA, during 1982 - 1985, was related to an excess concentration of heavy metal waste, especially of cadmium and chromium in sewage and river water. Both multiple sclerosis and myasthenia gravis were diagnosed by board-certified neurologists."

Myasthenia gravis, mentioned in the Ingalls research study, is a serious chronic disease of unknown cause which produces a defect in conduction of nerve impulses to muscles in the body. This causes progressive muscle weakness affecting many parts of the body. Fatigue is severe. People may have difficulty swallowing and trouble breathing if chest muscles are involved. Like MS, the cause is unknown and the disease progress can also have remissions and exacerbations.

Who exactly is T. Ingalls? Investigation led to the following information about T. Ingalls, MD. Theodore Ingalls was a Harvard graduate and professor emeritus of Boston University's Epidemiology Department. Dr. Ingalls is credited with developing the German measles vaccine. He is also said to have published more than 200 research papers. He spent a great deal of time in Galion, working with residents who tried for years to find out why so many people were stricken with MS. Dr. Ingalls was reported to be ill when the study was completed. This may explain why the ODH study results were not challenged.

Problems Found in the U.S. Public Health System

The need for a fully operational disease tracking network in this country should be clear, especially after reading about the many problems found in chronic disease cluster studies where no data on expected prevalence of a disease is available. Other studies claim that an increase of a disease in a community could not be determined due to lack of data on diseases in past years. A fully operational national disease tracking network could have all this information readily available. I know I have repeatedly brought this information to your attention. I truly feel that this information is vital to finding the cause and cure for many chronic diseases.

As mentioned in the beginning of the book, county health departments are typically not aware of a chronic disease cluster unless the disease cluster members contact them. The state health departments learn about a chronic disease cluster only if an individual contacts them or if the local health department contacts them. The CDC is the last to know, and only if the state health departments notifies them. There is no way of knowing how wide-spread chronic diseases really are if no one is collecting data and tracking them. If we knew where chronic disease clusters were located, we could compare environmental exposures and perhaps find a disease trigger or even a common cause for a disease. Investigations performed for disease clusters are hindered or delayed by missing information.

The need for a fully operation national disease tracking network is considered a top priority by public health advocacy organizations today. It is needed if we are ever going to control chronic disease epidemics. Federal agencies are concerned about the problems and weaknesses in our American

Chronic Disease / Pollution Connection

public health system, especially with the threat of bioterrorism. This is largely due to the efforts of over seventy public health advocacy groups such as Trust for Americas Health, Center for Health, Environment and Justice, the Environmental Health Network, and Physicians for Social Responsibility. A national disease tracking network could collect, analyze, and report data on the rate of chronic disease and the prevalent environmental factors and exposures.

The CDC funded a pilot study in 2002 (17.5 million dollars) to track diseases in a few states. In 2003 they awarded $28 million to 17 states, three cities and three schools of public health. The three Centers of Excellence involved in building the disease tracking system are Johns Hopkins University, Tulane University, and the University of California, Berkley. The total cost of the disease tracking network was estimated to be 275 million dollars a year, about $1 per American.

The American people can help the country reach its goal of a fully operational national disease tracking network by contacting their government representatives by letters, email, faxes, and phone calls. Contact information is available on the internet and at your public library.

The general public is reported to believe that chronic diseases are tracked throughout the country. Physicians also are said to believe most chronic disease tracking already occurs. The truth is that our public health infrastructure is not strong enough to do the job. Trust for Americas Health, in a 2003 report, addressed problems with public health agencies. The report titled, "Public Health Laboratories: Unprepared and Overwhelmed" came to the same conclusion. Health departments must have up-to-date laboratories to manage a widespread disease outbreak. An efficient computer system is necessary to manage a nationwide disease tracking network and any bioterrorism activities. These are lacking in many health departments.

Funding to health departments is reportedly diminishing, thus making it difficult to have up-to-date computers and other high-tech equipment. Also, there are no specific education requirements for many public health positions. Before we can have a fully operational disease tracking network, we have to build the infrastructure from the bottom up. That means starting with our local and state health departments.

Chapter 19

Mistakes Made and Lessons Learned By Disease Cluster Health Advocates

Lessons learned from the experiences of disease cluster members are listed below. These are provided in hopes that you can avoid repeating the same mistakes, and proceed more rapidly towards making your environment a cleaner place to live.

- Do not accept lack of action from your health departments and the EPA. Demand answers.
- Chronic disease clusters are everywhere. The numbers may be much higher than we can imagine.
- The goal of industry and big business is profit. Employee and community health are often low on their priority list.
- You can't assume that our health care agencies are willing and able to help you find a cause for your disease cluster.
- Science does not yet know the effects of low level toxic exposures over a prolonged period of time.
- Scientists know little about the effects of exposure to combinations of chemicals.

- You can stop industries from releasing excessive toxic chemicals into your environment if you know the laws and demand that the public agencies enforce them.
- Our national healthcare system is not operating efficiently and our tax dollars are often misused.
- Organized communities can have great power over corporations and government agencies. Know that one person can make a difference; don't wait for someone else to fight for you; or it may be too late.
- A national disease tracking network is vital to winning our battle against spreading chronic diseases and to managing bioterrorism.

Take notice of what is happening in your environment. Our environment is exposing us to uncontrolled toxic chemicals and causing chronic diseases all over the United States. Development of disease clusters is preventable. Toxic pollution can be controlled.

It is a sad commentary that we live in the most progressive country on earth but toxic environmental damage to Americans' health is not adequately controlled. The more communities get involved and ask the right questions, the more health officials will take notice and do the job our taxes pay them to do. Getting involved doesn't mean buying bottled water if you suspect your water source maybe contaminated, or organic vegetables if you learn that produce contains pesticide residue. We must stop the source of the pollution now for the sake of this generation and generations to come. Be proactive about stopping polluting industries from turning your neighborhood into a disease cluster, and you or a family member into a disease cluster statistic.

"The function of protecting and developing health must rank even above that of restoring it when it is impaired."
Hippocrates

Bibliography

American Cancer Society. "Cancer Facts and Figures 2005". <http://www.cancer.org/downloads/STT/CAFF2005f4PWSecured.pd>. 1 Apr. 2005.

Diegelman, Nathan. "Poison in the Grass: The Hazards And Consequences of Lawn Pesticides." The S.T.A.T.E Foundation. 19 Mar. 1998. <http://www.cqs.com/elawn.htm>. 2 Dec. 2004.

Dutzik, Tony, Jeremiah Baumann "Health Tracking and Disease Clusters, Lack of Data on Chronic Disease Incidence and Its Impact on Disease Cluster Investigations." PennEnvironment Research and Policy Center. Health Tracking and Disease Clusters. Sept. 2002. <www.pennenvironment.org/reports/healthtracking9_02.pdf>. Sept. 2003.

Frances Perkins. United States Secretary of Labor. U.S. Government Conference. Joplin Missouri. 23 April 1940. <http://historymatters.gmu.edu/d/128/.3>. Feb. 2004.

Harris, David T. "Immunotoxicology of JP8 Jet Fuel." Report number A447583. Arizona University ,Tucson. Nov. 2000.

Ingalls, Theodore MD. "Disease Clustering In Galion, Ohio 1982-1985." School of Public Health. Boston University School of Medicine. 10 Sept. 1989. <http://www.ncbi.nlm.nih.gov/entrez/query.fcgi?cmd=Retrieve&db=pubmed&dopt=Abstract&list_uids=2782299>. Sept. 2003.

Karp, Hal." A Town Divided: How a Cancer Threat is Tearing a Community Apart." Family Circle Magazine. August 2000.

Layco, Gambrelli M. and R. Wayne Ball. "Public Health Assessment. International Smelting and Refining Tooele, Tooele County, Utah". U.S. Department of Health. Center for Disease Control and Prevention .Agency For Toxic Substances and Disease Registry. 19 Oct. 2001. <www.atsdr.cdc.gov/HAC/PHA/internationalsmelting/isr_p1.html>. 28 Dec. 2004.

New York City, N.Y. Mount Sinai School of Medicine. Center for Children's Health and the Environment. Autism and Environmental Exposures. (n.d) <http://www.childenvironment.org/factsheets/autism.htm>. Mar. 2005.

PennEnvironment Research and Policy Center. Executive Summary. "Danger in the Air: Unhealthy Levels of Air Pollution in 2003". Sept. 2004. <http://www.pennenvironment.org/dangerintheair-9-04.html> Mar. 2005.

PennEnvironment Research and Policy Center. Executive Summary. "In Gross Violation: How Polluters are Flooding America's Waterways With Toxic Chemicals." October 2002. <http://www.pennevironment.org/ingrossviolation10-02.html>. Mar. 2004.

PennEnvironment Research and Policy Center. Executive Summary. "Toxic Releases and Health, a Review of Pollution Data and the Current Knowledge on the Health Effects of Toxic Chemicals." Jan. 2003. <http://www.pennenvironment.org/toxicsreleases1_03.html>. Nov. 2003.

Stewart, Sherri, Jessica King, Trevor Thompson, Carol Friedman, Phyllis Wingo. United States Center for Disease Control and Prevention. "Cancer Mortality Surveillance—United States, 1990-2000." Surveillance Summaries. 4 Jun. 2004.
<http://www.cdc.gov/mmwr/preview/mmwrhtml/ss5303a1.htm>. 9 Oct. 2004.

The Tennessean. "An Investigation Into Illnesses Around the Nations Nuclear Weapons Sites." Special Report For the Ill, Help Is Often Out of Reach. Feb. 1997.
<http://www.tennessean.com/sii/longterm/oakridge/part3/stories/nukmain.shtml>. Oct. 2003.

Toxic Action Center. "Toxics in Vermont: A Town-By-Town Profile." 13 Nov. 2003.
<http://www.toxicsaction.org/ToxicsReportVT04.pdf>. 15 Sept. 2004.

Trust For Americas Health. "Public Health Laboratories: Unprepared and Overwhelmed." June 2003.
<http://healthyamericans.org/reports/files/LabReport.pdf> 10 Aug. 2003.

Trust For Americas Health. "Childhood Cancer." Preventing Epidemics, Protecting People. Sept. 2003.
<httphealthyamericans.org/topics/index.php?TopicID=11>. Nov. 2004.

Trust For Americas Health. "How Well Are States Tracking Cancer?"(n.d)
<http://healthyamericans.org/state/cancergrade>. 3 Feb. 2004.

United States. Department of Health. Agency for Toxic Substances and Disease Registry. "Leukemia Cluster

Investigation in Fallon, Nevada." Media Announcement. 12 Feb. 2003.
<http://www.astdr.cdc.gov./NEWS/fallonei.html>. 4 May 2004.

United States. Department of Health. Agency for Toxic Substances and Disease Registry. "Motor Neuron Disease/ Amyotrophic Lateral Sclerosis Bexar County, (Kelly Air Force Base) Texas." 5 Mar. 2002.
<http://www.atsdr.cdc.gov/NEWS/alsreport.html>. 14 Oct. 2003.

United States. Department of Health. Agency for Toxic Substances and Disease Registry. "Public Health Statement for Jet Fuels JP-5 and JP-8." CAS # 80-08-20-6. Aug. 1998 <http://www.atsdr.cdc.gov/toxprofiles/phs76.html>. Apr. 2005.

United States. Department of Health. Center for Disease Control and Prevention. "Second National Report on Human Exposures to Environment Chemicals." 31 Jan. 2003.
<http://www.cdc.gov/exposurereport/2nd/>. 11 Sept. 2004.

United States. State of New Jersey Department of Health. Childhood Cancer Incidence Health Consultation. "A Review and Analysis of Cancer Registry Data 1979-1995. Dover Township (Ocean County) New Jersey." Sept. 1997. <http://www.state.nj.us/health/eoh/hhazweb/cansumm.pdf>. March 2003.

United States. Environmental Protection Agency. "Army Corps of Engineers Assists EPA in New Jersey Superfund Cleanup." (n.d.).
<http://www.epa.gov/superfund/news/acecleanup.htm>. Sept. 2002

United States. Environmental Protection Agency. "Asthma Facts." EPA 402-F-04-019. May 2005. <http://www.epa.gov/asthma/pdfs/asthma_fact_sheet_en.pdf>. 12 May 05.

United States Public Interest Research Group (USPIRG). Make Polluters Pay. "Health Effects of the Most Dangerous Substances Found at Superfund Sites." (n.d) <http://makepolluterspay.com/superfund.asp?id2=6208&id3=superfund&>. 25 Sept. 2004.

United States. State of Ohio Department of Health. Ohio Department of Health Release Study. "Marion County Leukemia Case Review" 26 Jul. 2001 <www.odh.state.oh.us/asset/iu_files/news072601.pdf >. 18 Jan. 2004.

United States. State of Ohio. Geauga County Health Department. Department Committee Meeting. "Middlefield Health Study Results." 20 May.2004. <http://www.geaugalink.com/townvill/mfdmins/vc040520.html>. 28 Jan. 2005.

United States. Department of Health. Agency for Toxic Substances and Disease Registry. "Asbestos Exposure in Libby Montana." ATSDR Involvement in Libby, Montana (n.d). <www.atsdr.cdc.gov/asbestos/asbestos_risks.html>. Aug. 2003.

United States. Department of Health. Agency for Toxic Substances and Disease Registry. "Mortality in Libby, Montana 1979-1998." Dec. 2000. <http://www.atsdr.cdc.gov/asbestos/mortalityinlibby.html>. 17 Jan. 2004.

United States. Department of Health. Agency for Toxic Substances and Disease Registry. "National Asbestos Exposure Review" ATSDR Health Consultation. 9Sept.2003. <http://www.atsdr.cdc.gov/naer/minotnd/hc.html>. 22 Aug 2004.

United States. Department of Health. Agency For toxic Substances and Disease Registry. "The Churchill County Leukemia Cluster Investigation in Fallon, Nev." Release Results of Environmental Exposure Pathway Fallon, Nevada. 12 Feb. 2003. <http://www.atsdr.cdc.gov/NEWS/fallonei.html>. 16 May 2004.

United States. Department of Health. Agency for Toxic Substances and Disease Registry. "Health Consultation. Potlatch Pulp Mill Lewiston, Nez Perce County Idaho." 19 Sept. 2000. <http://www.atsdr.cdc.gov/HAC/PHA/potlatch/ppm_toc.html>. 26 Oct. 2004.

United States. Department of Health. Agency for Toxic Substances and Disease Registry. "ALERT! Patterns of Metallic Mercury Exposure. How Does Mercury Affect Health." Updated Oct. 2003. <http://www.atsdr.cdc.gov/alerts/970626.html>. 11 Apr. 2004.

United States. Department of Health. Center for Disease Control and Prevention. Agency for Toxic Substances and Disease Registry. National Center for Environmental Health. "Environmental Etiologies Associated with Developmental Disabilities and the Brick Township, NJ Autism Cluster Investigation: Challenges in Identifying Environmental Etiologies." 25 Mar. 2004. <www.cdc.gov/nceh/tracking/presentations/thu/ses4B/f_bove.pdf>. 23 Mar. 2005.

United States. Department of Justice. Federal Registry. "Notice of Lodging a Consent Decree Under The Clean Air Act. 6 Nov.1998. Vol.63 N. 215." Page 60023-60024. <http://www.epa.gov/fedrgstr/EPA-AIR/1998/November/Day-06/a29707.htm>. Jun. 2004.

United States. Department of Health and Human Services. Center for Disease Control and Prevention. "Chronic Disease Overview." 15 Oct. 2004.
<http://www.cdc.gov/nccdphp/overview.htm> Apr. 2005.

United States. Department of Health and Human Services. Center for Disease Control and Prevention. "Birth Defects Frequently Asked Questions."(n.d)
<http://www.cdc.gov/ncbddd/bd/faq1.htm>. April 2005.

United States. Department of Health and Human Services. Center for Disease Control and Prevention. "Preventing and Controlling Cancer: Addressing the Nation's Second Leading Cause of Death." 2002.
<www.cdc.gov/nccdphp/aag/aag_dcpc.htm >. 12 Jan. 2005.

United States. Department of Health and Humans services. Center for Disease Control and Prevention. Second National Reprot on Expsure to Environmental Chemicals. "Body Burden". 2003.NCEH. Pub. No.02-0716.
<http://www.protectingourhealth.org/newscience/bodyburden/2003/2003-0131-CDC-bodyburden.htm>. May 2005

United States. .Department of Health and Human Services. Agency for Toxic Substances and Disease Registry. "Evaluating a Disease Cluster. Disease Clusters Case Studies." 2001.
<http://www.atsdr.cdc.gov/HEC/CSEM/cluster/evaluating.html>. Aug. 2002.

United States. .Department of Health and Human Services. Agency for Toxic Substances and Disease Registry . <u>Nez Perce Health Consultation</u> . "Evaluation of Air Exposure Potlatch Pulp Mill." 19 Sept. 2003. <http://www.atsdr.cdc.gov/HAC/PHA/potlatch/ppm_toc.html> . 9 Aug. 2004.

United States. Environmental Protection Agency. "Brick Township Landfill, New Jersey Ocean County." EPA District 2. EPA ID# NJD980505176. Feb. 2004 <http://www.epa.gov/region02/superfund/npl/0200540c.pdf>. Nov. 2004.

United States. Environmental Protection Agency. "Lead in Paint, Dust, and Soil." (n.d) <http://www.epa.gov/lead/leadinfo.htm>. May 2004.

United States. Environmental Protection Agency. National Lead Information Center Hotline. "Sources of Indoor Pollution. Lead." Updated 3 Mar. 2005. <http://www.epa.gov/iaq/lead.html>. 2 Oct. 2004.

United States. Environmental Protection Agency. <u>Endocrine Disruptors Screening Program.</u> "Endocrine Disruptors." <http://www.epa.gov/scipoly/oscpendo>. Mar. 2005.

United States. Environmental Protection Agency. "Waste Management."
<http://www.epa.nsw.gov.au/small_business/painters/wasteman.htm>. Feb. 2004.

United States. National Institute of Health. "Mercury Health Hazards". (n.d). <http://www.nih.gov/od/ors/ds/nomercury/health.htm>. May 2005

United.States. National Library of Medicine. National Institutes of Health. Specialized Information Services. "Household Products Database." <http://householdproducts.nlm.nih.gov>. April 2005.

Wagner,Gregory R. M.D. United States Department of Health and Human Services. Center for Disease Control and Prevention. "Work Place Exposure to Asbestos." Presentation Before the Senate Subcommittee on Environment and Public Works. Subcommittee on Superfund, Toxic Risk, and Waste Management 20 Jun.02
<http://epw.senate.gov/107th/Wagner_062002.htm>. 16 May 2005

Appendix A

Guide to Finding Help for Your Community's Environmental Health Problems

Computer addresses are included to access details about the following information. Some web sites may have changed. This occurs fairly often so you may have to browse the internet to pinpoint the information you want. *If you don't have access to a computer, your public library can help you find the information.*

Agency for Toxic Substances and Disease Registry (ATSDR)

The ATSDR is the lead public health agency responsible for implementing the health-related provisions of the Comprehensive Environmental Response, Compensation, and Liability Act of 1980 (CERCLA). ATSDR is responsible for assessing the presence and nature of health hazards at specific sites. ATSDR works closely with state agencies to carry out its mission of "preventing exposure to contaminants at hazardous waste sites and preventing adverse health effects. ATSDR provides funding and technical assistance for states to identify and evaluate environmental health threats to communities. These resources enable state and local health departments to further investigate environmental health concerns and educate communities. This is accomplished through cooperative agreements and grants". Their web site is www.atsdr.cdc.gov.

Center For Health Environment and Justice (CHEJ)

CHEJ is an environmental support group willing to assist you in combating the pollution in your environment. One example is the "Stop Dioxin Exposure Campaign", a national grassroots effort to eliminate dioxin and initiate a public debate on the role of government in protecting the health of the American people. CHEJ is a nonprofit, tax-exempt organization that provides organizing and technical assistance to grassroots community organizations nationwide. For more information on the "Stop Dioxin Exposure" campaign, visit this web site at www.safealternatives.org..

Communities for a Better Environment (CBE)

CBE is an environmental health and justice non profit organization promoting clean air, clean water, and the development of toxin-free communities in California. They provide grassroots activism, environmental research, and legal assistance within underserved urban communities. CBE directly equips residents impacted by industrial pollution with the tools to inform, monitor, and transform their immediate environment. More information can be found at www.cbecal.org.

Earthjustice

Earthjustice is a nonprofit public interest law firm. Their motto is "Even the Earth Needs a Good Lawyer." You can learn about your legal rights regarding environmental issues and about the activities of some communities fighting for their rights. Their website is www.earthjustice.org.

Environmental Working Group

This organization is comprised of scientists, engineers, policy experts, lawyers and computer programmers who provide reliable research findings on health and environmental issues. Their computer site is www.ewg.org.

Freedom of Information Act (FOIA)

Enacted in 1966, the FOIA gives any person the right to access federal records (except for nine exemptions and three law enforcement record exclusions). For specifics and sample request letters, please go to the National Institute of Standards and Technology internet site is www.nist.gov/admin/foia/foia.htm.

You can also use the FOIA to access your local government records. Examples of information you might want to access in your communities would be records from your closed city council meetings and your school board meeting minutes. Remember to state that you are requesting information under the Freedom of Information Act.

National Institute of Health (NIH)

The NIH provides excellent information on all diseases and conditions. Here you can learn about research on many of these conditions. Their web site is www.nih.gov.

The NIH National Library of Medicine is a good source of information on 650 topics that cover conditions, diseases and wellness. They also provide information about prescription and over the counter drugs.

The NIH also provides lists of household products that can have harmful effects on our health. Check their website for lists of household products and chemicals found in each product. Just about every product is covered. One surprising finding was that one of the most popular laundry detergents on the market today contains chemicals that are known to cause lung cancer.
http://householdproducts.nlm.nih.gov.

Physicians for Social Responsibility

This organization provides very well-written and easily-understood information for citizens and healthcare providers. You will find detailed reports on such subjects as toxic substances, children's health, air pollution, chronic disease and the environment, and safe drinking water. Their website is www.envirohealthaction.org.

Scorecard

Scorecard is respected for its accurate pollution information. The data is taken from scientific sources, and state and federal regulatory agencies. They provide health information on chemical exposures that are suspected of adversely affecting your health. You will find information on just about any chronic disease and the corresponding suspected chemical exposures. Scorecard provides statistics for most every town or city in the United States. The Scorecard website for information, www.scorecard.org is very user friendly! You will be surprised by how much you can learn about your community.

Sierra Club

The Sierra Club is one of the largest, most influential grassroots environmental organizations. The organization provides information on the environment and environmental law. Their website is www.sierraclub.org.

The Environmental Protection Agency (EPA)

The U.S.EPA is good source for information on many topics that a health advocate would find useful. Examples of some topics are acid rain, global warming, hazardous waste, ozone, pesticides, and pollution in your community. Superfund sites and Brownfield are under EPA jurisdiction as are the Clean Air Act and the Clean Water Act. It is very helpful if you understand how these areas are supposed to be operated by your EPA, so you can remind them when they fail to enforce laws. The U.S.EPA website is at www.epa.gov.

An EPA office is located near you. Each state has district EPA offices covering the state. These districts are numbered to determine the communities covered by each office. For example, Wellington, Ohio is covered by the Ohio EPA District 5 Office. You must make an appointment to visit your EPA district office to look up information on industries. Under the Freedom of Information Act, you should have access to every report covering the history of each industry and any pollution law noncompliance.

The Toxic Release Inventory (TRI) is also available to the public through the U.S.EPA website. You will find the reported names and amounts of chemicals in your communities that are released yearly into your air and water.

Trust for Americas Health (TFAH)

TFAH is a very successful, nonprofit, non partisan organization. Their mission is dedicated to saving lives by protecting the health of every community and working to make disease prevention a national priority. They are responsible for the passage of important government public health legislation. They support public health advocacy and are willing to help you fight for your community's health. TFAH provides research data on your states environmental efforts or lack of efforts to track diseases. Contact TFAH via their website at www.healthyamericans.org.

Appendix B

Glossary of Acronyms

Most businesses and all federal agencies identify themselves using the first initial of each word in their title. This can be maddening to someone unfamiliar with the practice. There are only a few that you will see repeatedly used in this book. Hopefully once you learn them it will become easier. English grammar rules require their use in this way in this book.

ALL	Acute Lymphocytic Leukemia
ALS	Amyotrophic Lateral Sclerosis
AML	Acute Myelogenous Leukemia
ATSDR	U.S. Agency for Toxic Substances and Disease Control
AWARES	Abington, Weymouth and Rockland Environmental Studies
BEHS	Bureau of Environmental Health and Safety
CDC	Center for Disease Control and Prevention
CRVF	Concerned River Valley Families
EPA	Environmental Protection Agency
FIST	Families In Search of Truth

FOIA	Freedom of Information Act
LCHD	Lorain County Health Department
MCS	Multiple Chemical Sensitivity
MS	Multiple Sclerosis
NCEH	National Center for Environmental Health
NHL	Non Hodgkin's Lymphoma
NIH	National Institute of Health
NPCR	National Program of Cancer Registries
ODH	Ohio Department of Health
OEPA	Ohio Environmental Protection Agency
PCBS	polychlorinated biphenyls
PIRG	Public Information Research Group
PSR	Physicians for Social Responsibilities
PPM	Parts per million
TCE	Trichloroethylene
TFAH	Trust For Americas Health
TRI	Toxic Release Inventory
TVA	Tennessee Valley Authority

US EPA	United States Environmental Protection Agency
US PIRG	United States Public Interest Research Group

Appendix C

Health Effects of the Most Toxic Substances Found at Superfund Sites

This reference for the most toxic substances found at superfund sites and their affects on health is provided by the U.S. Public Information Group.

"Link to the Agency for Toxic Substances and Disease Registry (ATSDR) Most Dangerous Substances: http://www.atsdr.cdc.gov/toxpro2.html.

Link to Scorecard's search engine for chemicals: http://www.scorecard.org/chemical-profiles.

ARSENIC

Health Effects: Arsenic is known to cause cancer of the lungs, bladder, and skin. Arsenic is also linked to cancer of the liver, kidney, colon and nasal passages, and to a variety of non-cancer health effects, including heart disease, diabetes, adverse impacts on the immune system, lungs, and gastrointestinal track, and thickening and discoloration developmental impacts. Scorecard | ATSDR

LEAD

Health Effects: Lead can damage almost every organ and system in the human body, especially the immune and reproductive systems, and can cause heart disease and kidney damage. Lead is exceptionally damaging to the central nervous system, particularly in children where it can cause brain damage. Lead has can also decrease IQ scores, slow growth, and cause hearing problems in infants or young children. Scorecard | ATSDR

MERCURY

Health Effects: Mercury can cause brain and kidney damage, and poses an especially high risk of adverse neurological development of fetuses. Scorecard | ATSDR

VINYL CHLORIDE

Health Effects: Vinyl chloride can cause cancer, and may damage the liver and immune and nervous systems. Scorecard |ATSDR

POLYCHLORINATED BUPHENYLS (PCBs)

Health Effects: PCBs can cause cancer and adverse developmental impacts. These impacts may include lowered IQ and behavioral problems such as Attention Deficit Disorder. PCBs are also linked to adverse reproductive impacts, including low birth weight, damage to the immune system. Scorecard | ATSDR

BENZENE

Health Effects: Benzene causes cancer, and adverse developmental and reproductive impacts. Benzene may also cause damage to the immune, respiratory, endocrine and cardiovascular system. Scorecard | ATSDR

CADMIUM

Health Effects: Cadmium causes cancer and adverse reproductive and developmental impacts. It may also damage the lungs, kidneys and digestive track, and has been linked to weakening of the immune system and human skeletal system. Scorecard | ATSDR

BENZO (A) PYRENE

Health Effects: Benzo (a) pyrene, a Polycyclic Aromatic Hydrocarbon (PAH), causes cancer and may damage to the developmental, immune and respiratory systems. Scorecard | ATSDR

POLYCYCLIC AROMATIC HYDROCARBONS (PAH)

Health Effects: Polycyclic Aromatic Hydrocarbons (PAHs) are a group of over 100 different chemicals formed during the incomplete burning of coal, oil and gas, garbage, or other organic substances. Some PAHs cause cancer, and may adversely affect the reproductive and immune systems. Scorecard | ATSDR

CHLOROFORM

Health effects: Chloroform can cause cancer, and may damage the liver, kidneys, and endocrine and respiratory systems. Chloroform may also cause birth defects and miscarriages. Scorecard | ATSDR

DDT, P, P1

Health Effects: DDT can cause cancer and adverse developmental and reproductive impacts. DDT may also damage the liver and central nervous system, causing excitability, tremors, and seizures in people. Scorecard | ATSDR

AROCLOR 1254

Health Effects: Aroclor 1254 is a form of polychlorinated biphenyl (PCB). PCBs can cause cancer and adverse developmental impacts. These impacts may include lowered IQ and behavioral problems such as Attention Deficit Disorder. PCBs are also linked to adverse reproductive impacts, including low birth weight, damage to the immune system. Scorecard | ATSDR

AROCLOR 1260

Health Effects: Aroclor 1260 is a form of polychlorinated biphenyl (PCB). PCBs can cause cancer and adverse developmental impacts. These impacts may include lowered

IQ and behavioral problems such as Attention Deficit Disorder. PCBs are also linked to adverse reproductive impacts, including low birth weight and damage to the immune system. Scorecard | ATSDR

TRICHLOROETHYLENE

Health Effects: Trichloroethylene can cause cancer and may damage the nervous system, liver, and lungs. It may also cause adverse reproductive and developmental impacts, and damage to the cardiovascular and immune system. Scorecard | ATSDR

DIBENZO (A, H) ANTHRACENE

Health Effects: Dibenzo (a, h) anthracene is a Polycyclic Aromatic Hydrocarbon (PAH) suspected of causing cancer. PAHs are a group of over 100 different chemicals formed during the incomplete burning of coal, oil and gas, garbage, or other organic substances. Some PAHs cause cancer, and may adversely affect the reproductive and immune systems. Scorecard | ATSDR

DIELDRIN

Health Effects: Dieldrin causes cancer and damage to the nervous system. Dieldrin may also damage the cardiovascular, immune, reproductive, and respiratory systems. Low exposure can cause headaches, dizziness, vomiting, irritability, and uncontrolled muscle movements. Scorecard | ATSDR

HEXAVALENT CHROMIUM

Health Effects: Hexavalent chromium (or chromium (VI) causes cancer and may damage the kidney and liver. Large exposures of hexavalent chromium can cause death. Scorecard |ATSDR

CHLORDANE

Health Effects: Chlordane causes cancer and may damage the nervous, cardiovascular, reproductive, and digestive system and the liver. Low doses of chlordane can also cause headaches, irritability, confusion, weakness, vision problems, vomiting, stomach cramps, diarrhea, and jaundice. Ingesting large amounts can cause convulsions and death. Scorecard | ATSDR

HEXACHLOROBUTADIENE

Health Effects: Hexachlorobutadiene may cause cancer and damage to cardiovascular system, and kidneys and liver. It may also cause adverse developmental and reproductive impacts. Scorecard | ATSDR"

Printed in the United States
36892LVS00002B/31-57